"I Want to See"

Vision for the World

Published in 2000 by
World Eye Surgeons Society
c/o Singapore National Eye Centre
11 Third Hospital Avenue, Singapore 168751
and
World Scientific Publishing Co. Pte Ltd
P O Box 128, Farrer Road, Singapore 912805

USA office
Suite 1B, 1060 Main Street, River Edge,
NJ 07661

UK office
Shelton Street, Covent Garden,
London WC2H 9HE

Vision for the World, 1st Edition, 1996
"I Want to See": Vision for the World, 2nd Edition, 2000

World Eye Surgeons Society
World Scientific Publishing Co. Pte Ltd

ISBN 981 02 4311 (hardcover)
ISBN 981 02 4312 X

Book code 4428

Design by SinKho Advertising and Design

Printed in Singapore

"I Want to See"

Vision for the World

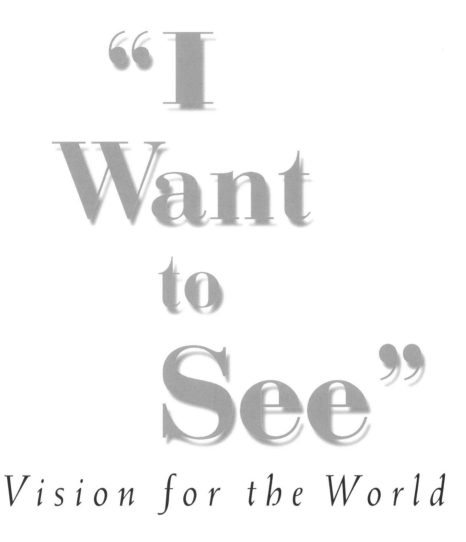

WRITERS AND EDITORS

Ang Beng Chong, Adrian Koh, Julian Theng, Lee Shu Yen,
Chan Poh Geok, Charity Wai, Julie Goh, Leona Lo

Author of *Vision for the World*, 1st edition
Arthur SM Lim

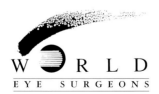

WORLD
EYE SURGEONS

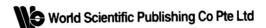 World Scientific Publishing Co Pte Ltd

"I Want to See"

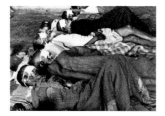

Contents

Contents

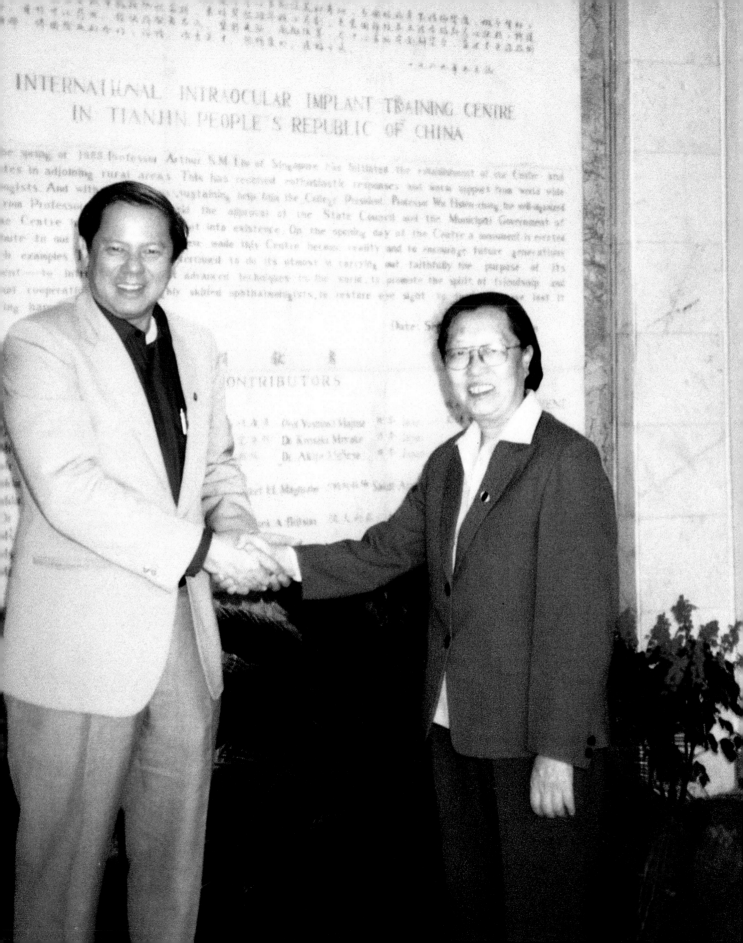

Dedication

Search our hearts: just how many blind patients have we, as eye surgeons, restored normal vision to? More than 1,000 in a lifetime? Imagine the overwhelming achievement and joy of restoring normal vision to 120,000 people blind from cataract.

As the Founding Director of the International Intraocular Implant Training Centre (IIITC), Tianjin, China, Professor Yuan is planning to restore normal vision to 1,000,000. Although a seemingly insurmountable task, Professor Yuan Jia-Qin is a remarkable ophthalmologist who is well on her way to achieving this target.

Under the auspices of her leadership, the IIITC, which she herself initiated and established, has taught 2,250 ophthalmologists modern cost-effective ECCE and PCI under the operating microscope.

It can be said that in the prevention of blindness, Professor Yuan is the leading light in our fight for sight. Indeed, she is the eye surgeon of the 20th century.

Foreword

Prof. Dr. G.O.H. Naumann, *PRESIDENT, INTERNATIONAL COUNCIL OF OPHTHALMOLOGY*

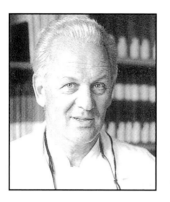

It is indeed a privilege and a great pleasure for me to write this foreword for "I Want to See", the 2nd Edition of "Vision for the World".

As we cross the threshold into the 3rd millennium, I believe that ophthalmologists around the world should unite to pursue a global initiative to champion the importance of vision and to alleviate the misery of blindness of their fellowmen.

The Tianjin Eye Centre described in this book is an excellent example of how ophthalmologists have come together to successfully tackle the major blinding condition of cataracts afflicting over 5 million people in the People's Republic of China. My colleague and dear friend, Prof Arthur Lim, is to be congratulated for his vision and foresight some ten years ago in initiating and sponsoring the establishment of this centre, and, at the same time, pushing for reforms and the teaching of the modern technique of cataract surgery with intraocular lens implantation.

His partner in this sterling effort to combat mass cataract blindness is Prof Yuan Jia-Qin, an energetic and totally dedicated ophthalmologist in Tianjin, who at the age of 70 took up the colossal challenge and achieved remarkable results. The Centre has trained over 2,250 ophthalmologists from all parts of China, performed over 120,000 cataract implant surgeries with its network of affiliated hospitals and has set a further target of performing 1 million cataract implant surgeries with other collaborating centres in China in the next 5 years.

This book, "I Want to See", contains a powerful message that ophthalmologists have a unique opportunity to come together to fulfil their noble mission of bringing vision and hope to the victims of curable blindness and of making a difference to mankind.

I am confident that ophthalmologists around the world will respond resoundingly to Arthur Lim's call for unity and global cooperation.

Gottfried O. H. Naumann

Gottfried Naumann
President of International Council of Ophthalmology
January 18, 2000

Preface

Vision for the World

Why a New Edition?

The main reason is the positive reviews we received from numerous leading lights in ophthalmology. Some of their comments are attached.

Next, this volume aims to mark the changes in approach of some world organisations; notably, WHO, since the 1st Edition. After more than ten years of disagreement, there has been a shift from ICCE to ECCE with PCI. This shift is historic because ICCE gives poor visual results compared to the restoration of normal vision with ECCE and implants. I thank these international organisations, in particular, WHO, for their efforts because I know how difficult it is for large organisations to change direction.

We hope that within 10 years, blindness from cataract will be controlled and reversed, especially since new blinding conditions — such as diabetic retinopathy and glaucoma — are already emerging.

The Cynosure of Modern Eye Centres: the Tianjin Eye Centre, People's Republic of China

When the prestigious Tianjin Eye Centre, People's Republic of China, successfully trains 2,250 eye surgeons in low-cost, modern cataract surgical techniques, and restores normal vision to 120,000 patients, with plans to attain the impressive figure of 1,000,000 — the world should acknowledge its innovative and efficacious methods. Its Medical Director, Prof Yuan Jia-Qin, should also be recognised as a world leader in ophthalmology in the 20th century.

The Historic Decision of the World Bank

We must also acknowledge and recognise the historic decision of the World Bank, under the direction of its President Mr James D Wolfensohn and his team, to issue a US$188-million loan to India. The aim is to teach and perform ECCE and PCI so as to restore normal vision to the millions blind from cataract in India. I take this opportunity to congratulate the World Bank and to thank the Indian government for their efforts towards cataract blindness prevention in India.

About the Book

At the same time, I feel there are still many outstanding problems yet to be resolved. The collection of articles, ideas, thoughts, correspondences, interviews and controversies in this book aims to address such concerns. This publication will also address the eye-care dilemma affecting governments, WHO, NGOs, eye doctors and patients, and will, I hope, prompt them to adopt major reforms in eye-care services in the coming millennium.

I have humbly taken on the danger of telling unwelcome truths, as I believe that we would not be able to rise up to the challenges of this exciting century if facts are submerged and vital questions are left unanswered.

It is sad that the resistance to change has been so intense, and that several leading international ophthalmologists — who were also close personal friends of many years — were concerned and promptly advised me to drop these issues for fear that powerful individuals and organisations might move against me.

I have asked myself daily whether I should simply look up to the European, American and Japanese leaders for their intellectual and scientific opinions on what is required in the developing nations and not challenge their failure to introduce ECCE and PCI, their reluctance to support training centres in the People's Republic of China and the unequal representation of developing nations in the International Council of Ophthalmology (ICO) and the Academia Ophthalmologica Internationalis.

I thank a dedicated team of editors and ophthalmologists who designed, researched and came up with the concept for this edition. I am also grateful to them for painstakingly vetting the manuscripts. Their support has strengthened my decision not to be cowed into silence by threats or fear.

It is wise to discuss these issues openly even if they may generate disagreement. The controversies which may be raised in this publication are not meant to sow discord, but to stimulate progress. If we are to progress, it is essential that we discuss important reforms for a better tomorrow.

When issues are complex, we must always remind ourselves of Asia's celebrated Nobel Laureate, Rabindranath Tagore, who stated that "If we are not open, the door to the truth will be shut."

We also have to look into the growing importance of good vision for everyone, especially for our ageing population. The growing demand for quality eye-care, together with escalating health costs and the proliferation of costly, high-technology will force changes in ophthalmic practice and training. If we are to provide quality vision for the world in this coming millennium, major reforms are inevitable.

"I Want to See" is a historic testimony of the world's battle against mass cataract blindness. It attests to the unwavering spirit with which ophthalmologists and their supporters from around the world have devoted themselves to this worthy cause.

The *Introduction* chronicles the birth of modern ophthalmology in Singapore and throughout the world. From its humble beginnings, ophthalmology in Singapore has flourished to attain world-class status. Today, the Singapore National Eye Centre (SNEC) is the proud standard-bearer of local and international ophthalmology.

I Want to See, first published in the Hong Kong Journal of Ophthalmology, October 1997, Vol. 1, No. 3, echoes the plaintive cries of millions of blind cataract victims around the world. Their suffering will only cease when we acknowledge ECCE with PCI as the choice method for cataract surgery.

With rapid political and economic progress in Asia, there will be reforms in the management of major blinding conditions in this part of the world. *Ophthalmology in Asia Awakes!* illustrates the spectacular success of ophthalmology in Asia, and holds up the 1990 26th International Congress of Ophthalmology, held in Singapore, as a stark indication that Asia has awoken. Yet Asia's awakening brings with it the attendant problems of escalating costs and rising expectations. How should ophthalmologists confront these problems in the 21st century? This is addressed in *The Dilemma of Ophthalmic Changes Spreads to Asia*, Editorial, American Journal of Ophthalmology, Vol. 123, June 1999.

A rising star in Asian ophthalmology is the International Intraocular Implant Training Centre (IIITC) in Tianjin, China, which has established itself as a model eye centre for the world to follow. *Tianjin Centre: A Model for the World to Follow* explores the secrets behind the centre's spectacular success.

Under the beneficent leadership of Professor Yuan Jia-Qin, the Tianjin Centre has trained 2,250 eye surgeons and has restored normal vision to 120,000 blind cataract victims. This points to the crucial role that ophthalmologists play in the battle against mass blindness, as highlighted in the *First Susruta Memorial Lecture: Increasing Importance of Eye Surgeons in Mass*

Preface

Blindness – A Megatrend (1993). Naturally, the ophthalmologists must be competent, as skilled eye surgeons are the best guarantee of quality surgical outcome. The importance of *Quality Outcome* was stressed in the prestigious Barraquer Gold Medal Lecture – *Towards Perfect Outcome in Cataract Surgery: The Eye Surgeon's Role* (1997).

As the battle against mass cataract blindness raged on, I was interviewed by the Television Corporation of Singapore (TCS) on 8 May 1996. They were intrigued by my persistence in advocating the use of ECCE with PCI as the principal means of providing *Quality Cataract Surgery in Rural Asia in the 21st Century*.

This was swiftly followed by an editorial in the American Journal of Ophthalmology in October 1996, Vol. 122: *Eye Surgeons – Seize the Opportunity*, published in conjunction with the American Academy of Ophthalmology Centennial Meeting.

But the efforts of ophthalmologists alone are not enough. The various world organisations must recognize and endorse the benefits of quality surgical techniques before ophthalmology can advance. The resistance to change of certain world organizations was highlighted in the 1997 interview on *Changing World Opinion?* conducted by Dr Ronald Yeoh, Visiting Consultant at the Singapore National Eye Centre.

WORLDEYES, a uniquely Asian initiative, is a heartening example of what ophthalmologists can achieve with dedication and unity. Through the concerted efforts of 1,000 volunteer eye surgeons, 5 cataract implant training centres have been established in China under the aegis of WORLDEYES. Numerous teaching courses and life surgery demonstrations have also been conducted at these centres by leading ophthalmologists — all volunteers of WORLDEYES.

Amidst the whirl and frenzy of the 21st century, the spectres of escalating costs and rising expectations will continue to haunt ophthalmologists around the world. Are we prepared to reform? For ophthalmology to sally forth triumphantly in this millennium, we need to imbibe the sparkling inventiveness and commitment of Asian ophthalmologists like Professor Yuan Jia-Qin (China), the late Professor Zhang Xiao-lou (China), the late Jose Rizal (the Philippines) — who was executed for his nationalist ideals — and Susruta, the father of ophthalmology in about 1000 BC. Further, we have to endorse and applaud the brilliant achievements of outstanding young Asian ophthalmologists like Professor Dennis Lam (Hong Kong), Associate Professor Vivian Balakrishnan (Singapore) and Assistant Professor Wong Tien Yin (Singapore). We must cultivate their talents and create opportunities for them to propel ophthalmology to higher stratospheres. In the coming years, the ophthalmic world will resound with the triumphs of a new generation of ophthalmologists.

Arthur Lim
Founder President
World Eye Surgeons Society

Reviews of World Leaders
"Vision for the World"
First Edition

THE WAY TO GO

"I certainly believe that with the availability of relatively inexpensive intraocular lenses and the superior educational programs, such as you are providing, you will soon remove any controversy that ECCE and PCI is 'the way to go' in people's minds."

Professor Bruce Spivey,
M.D.:Secretary-General, International Council of Ophthalmology; United States

BEAUTIFULLY PREPARED

"I have thoroughly enjoyed reviewing your compilation of information and your strong appeal for an international effort to overcome this important cause of blindness. This informative and beautifully prepared volume is a result of your commitment to provide the best possible eye care for people throughout the world."

Professor Bradley R Straatsma,
M.D.: Editor-in-Chief, American Journal of Ophthalmology; United States.

CRUSADER

"I'm absolutely enthusiastic about the leadership you are personally providing to our never ending crusade – there are not many crusaders such as you! I continue to be amazed by all your accomplishments, and of course, by your willingness to be innovative and go the full hundred yards."

Professor Alfred Sommer,
M.D.: Dean, School of Hygiene and Public Health, Johns Hopkins University; United States.

DEDICATION & IDEALS

"You are a living example of what dedication, ideals, and knowledge can contribute to humanity."

Professor Benjamin Boyd,
M.D.:President, Academia Ophthalmologica Internationalis; Panama.

MASTERFULLY ORGANISED

"My most sincere congratulations! It is really a tremendous endeavour you have accomplished. I want to express my willingness to offer my cooperation for this extraordinary humanitarian, and masterfully organised, medical programme."

Professor Enrique Malbran,
M.D.: Director, Malbran Ophthalmology Centre; Buenos Aires, Argentina.

DELIGHT

"I have read your work with delight because it will be useful in the programs that the Fundacion Oftalmologica Nacional currently use to prevent blindness in Columbia."

Professor Alvaro Rodriguez,
M.D.: Director, National Ophthalmological Foundation; Columbia.

MAGNIFICENT

"I always read your letters with a lift of heart and your 'Vision for the World' concept is inspiring. You are really doing a magnificent job in promoting a rational global programme to reduce this needless form of disability, affecting such a multitude of people."

Sir John Wilson,
C.B.E.: Chairman, IMPACT; Brighton, United Kingdom.

MASTERPIECE

"You did it again. I admire your enthusiasm in your battle against cataract blindness. Your monograph on 'Vision for the World' is a masterpiece and well worth your effort. It contains a lot of information for those who will follow your steps."

Professor JJ De Laey,
M.D.: Professor and Chairman, Department of Ophthalmology, University of Ghent, Belgium.

Reviews of World Leaders
"Vision for the World"
First Edition

VERY IMPORTANT

"The control of world blindness is now in the hands of eye surgeons of the world, not only in University Professors and well known Scientists, but also in the hands of all young surgeons all around the world. Let us take this opportunity to make the world a better place. What you are doing to help the world's blind is very important, and I deeply appreciate your efforts."

Professor Gabriel Coscas,
M.D.: Professor and Chairman, Eye University Clinic of Creteil, University of Paris XII, France.

UNDERSTANDING

"I hope you will still, for a long time, strengthen ophthalmology links in the East. It is thanks to you that in the West, we get a better understanding of all these very complex problems."

Professor Pierce Almaric,
M.D.: Dean, School of Hygiene and Public Health, Johns Hopkins University, United States.

GREAT ADMIRATION

"It is a beautiful book about a magnificent project that will make so vast a difference to the lives of so many — 40 million — fellow humans. You deserve the warmest accolade and great admiration that will certainly come your way."

Professor Lim Pin,
Vice-Chancellor, National University of Singapore, Singapore.

GREAT ASSET

"Thank you very much for your book, 'Vision for the World'. I was very inspired by it. You are a great asset to Singapore and to the World."

ProfessorTommy Koh,
Director, The Institute of Policy Studies, Singapore.

AT THE FOREFRONT

"I must congratulate you for your fine efforts to put Asian Ophthalmology at the forefront. I agree with your views entirely and you have my support all the way."

Professor S Selverajah,
M.D. : Past-President, Asia-Pacific Academy of Ophthalmology, Malaysia.

INSPIRATION

"Vision for the World" will be an inspiration to any eye surgeon in Asia who reads it. It is going to occupy an important place in our library. Please accept my best wishes for a very very long working life. You are very much needed.

Dr P N Nagpal,
M.D.: Eye Research Centre and Retina Foundation, Ahmedabad, India.

FULLY AGREE

"I fully agree with you that cataract blindness, by the turn of the century, will be the commonest and one of the most serious disabilities afflicting millions of otherwise normal individuals. The happy news is that we can restore their normal vision through ECCE and PCIOL."

Professor M Daud Khan,
M.D.: President, Asia-Pacific Academy of Ophthalmology, Pakistan.

OUTSTANDING

"It is outstanding, the work that you have done in Tianjin, and the work that has also been done in Bangladesh."

Professor Hugh R Taylor,
M.D.: Professor, Department of Ophthalmology, University of Melbourne, Australia.

HUMANITARIAN

"It is both a scientific and humanitarian public service work. I am ready to give a hand any time you ask me to do so. I am determined to call on other colleagues who are also able to promote the procedure all over Egypt."

Professor Abdel Latif Siam,
M.D.:Professor, Cairo, Egypt.

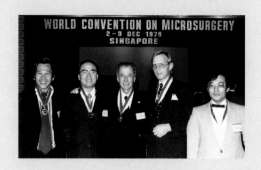

Introduction
From Dreams to Actions

Chapter 1

Introduction:
From Dreams to Actions

"That an eye surgeon from the People's Republic of China, Professor Yuan Jia-Qin, has transformed our dreams into action, marks a historic chapter in the 20th century."

Dreams that shatter the world's complacency, that fire mankind's imagination and that grapple with contemporary crises are rare and worthy dreams. But even such dreams would be rendered hollow if they are not acted on. When we dream of the wonders of modern ophthalmology for everyone, everywhere, it is wrong to just dream, listen or observe, and let ideas idle in silence. If ideas to improve ophthalmology are to develop and if we are to use science and technology to overcome the destructive forces of nature, then the obstacles to better eye-care for everyone must be eradicated.

For centuries, we have known that ideas for important changes can be disturbing or even frightening — they will stimulate the imagination of everyone and will also displease those in charge. But major ideas for quality, for progress, for equality and for justice have always attracted resistance. If these ideas are not transformed rapidly into action, is there

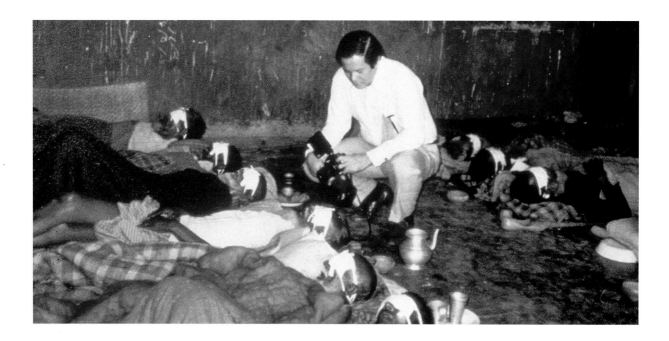

Cataract eye camp in one of the poor neglected areas of Bangladesh.

hope for a wonderful future for eye-care? Ideas sometimes appear wrong and sometimes, unfortunately, are deliberately made to appear wrong, and their supporters criticized by those in charge. But if these are ideas which genuinely benefit society, they will eventually resurface and provoke our social conscience again. Besides, the resistance to change itself frequently fans the fire of public interest, and focuses attention on the ideas. In the words of France's foremost writer, Victor Hugo:

> *"An invasion of armies can be resisted; but not an idea whose time has come."*

Asia's spectacular transition from dreams to action occurred in the 1960s, with the emergence of numerous ophthalmic groups and the globalization of Asia's contribution to the prevention of blindness. In 1960, the Asia-Pacific Academy of Ophthalmology (APAO) was formed. In 1964, at the Second Congress of the APAO held in Melbourne, Australia, in a paper entitled *Prevention of Blindness in Singapore*, the importance of blindness and its prevention was emphasized.

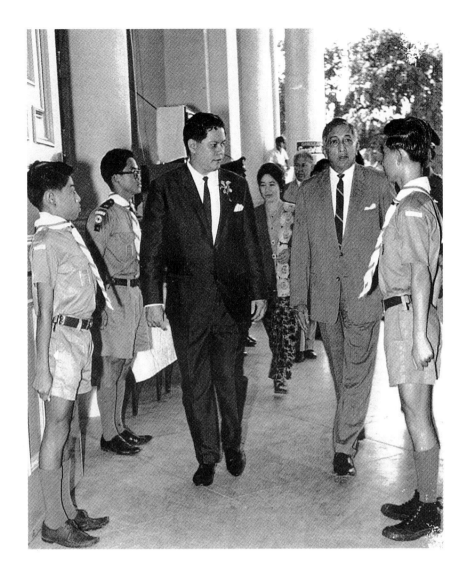

Author with Yusof Ishak,
President, Republic of Singapore.

The glittering expansion of ophthalmic activities in Asia continued unabated. In 1965, the Singapore Association for the Blind (SAB) expanded its international activities. The President of the Republic of Singapore, Mr Yusof Ishak — who was also the Patron of the association — and his wife, Puan Noor Aisha, strongly supported the association's activities.

During the 1970s, Sir John Wilson founded the International Agency for the Prevention of Blindness (IAPB) and multiple moves were made to

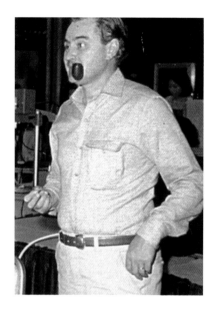
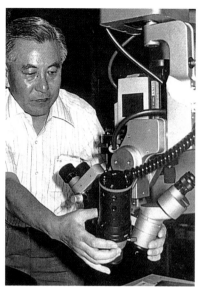
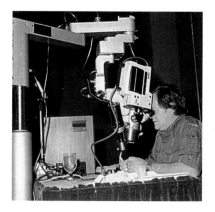

Microsurgery teaching courses.
From left: Noel Rice (UK), Saiichi Mishima (Japan)
and Dick Galbraith (Australia)

improve conditions for eye-care in the developing nations. One great achievement was the creation of worldwide interest in blindness and its prevention.

The quality of eye surgery in Asia improved dramatically when microsurgery was taught to hundreds of eye surgeons throughout Asia, with Singapore as the international teaching centre. The World Convention on Microsurgery (1979) and the International Workshop on Microsurgery (1981), in conjunction with The Royal Australasian College of Surgeons and The Royal Australasian College of Ophthalmologists respectively, both took place in Singapore. This was possible because leading ophthalmic microsurgeons came to Singapore to help run the numerous microsurgical courses. Asia is indebted to Prof Joaquin Barraquer (Spain), Prof Ian Constable (Australia), Dr Dick Galbraith (Australia), Prof Saiichi Mishima (Japan), Dr Thomas Moore (USA) and Dr Noel Rice (United Kingdom).

In the 1982 International Congress of Ophthalmology in San Francisco, it was estimated that less than 2% of the world's population in the developing nations had access to modern eye-care such as microsurgery, laser treatment, vitrectomy and fundal fluorescein angiography. In the poorer developing countries, the problem was even more basic. The major preventable and curable causes of blindness in these countries included cataract, blinding malnutrition (keratomalacia), blinding infection (trachoma), corneal ulcers and onchocerciasis. The number of blind in the world was expected to get worse as the number of patients suffering from cataract increased with the increased lifespan.

The International Ophthalmological Academic Meeting in Guangzhou, 1985, attracted numerous leading lights in ophthalmology who gathered to pay homage to Professor Eugene Chan for his outstanding contribution to ophthalmology in China. Key issues in ophthalmology were addressed at this prestigious meeting.

Why are there millions blind from cataract when the condition can simply be cured by extracting the opaque lens? The reasons for the failure of the eye-care delivery system are complex as they are

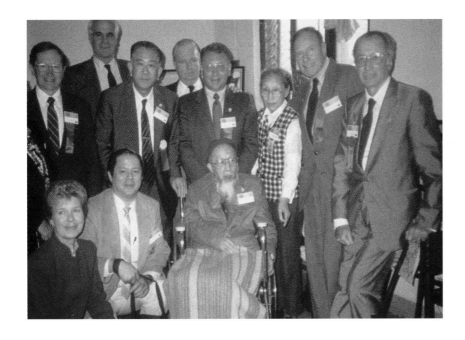

From left, standing: Bradley Straatsma (USA), David Paton (USA), Akira Nakajima (Japan), the late Edward Norton (USA), Bruce Spivey (USA), Winifred Mao (China), Carl Kupfer (USA) and Joaquin Barraquer (Spain). From left, sitting: Ruth Straatsma (USA), Arthur Lim (Singapore) and Eugene Chen (Guangzhou, China).

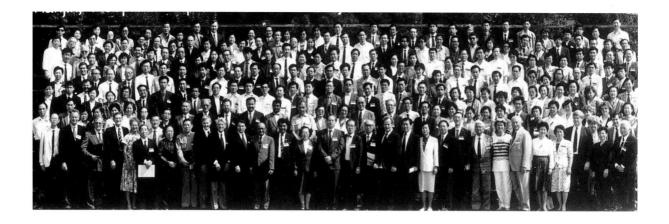

A group picture of the 1st International Meeting of the Tianjin International Intraocular Implant Training Centre attended by about 200 participants.

dependent on the politico-socioeconomic and cultural situation of the country involved. In the Holmes Lecture (1987), I emphasized that given the spread of affluence and modern technology in the wealthier developing countries, ophthalmologists in Asia would be in an excellent position to lead and to ensure high standards of care for patients suffering from cataract and other major blinding conditions.

A major reason why the control of cataract has been poor is due to the lack of leadership from eye surgeons. After all, patients blind from cataract require surgery, and surgery requires competent eye surgeons. The problem intensified when it was clear 20 years ago that intraocular implant following extracapsular cataract extraction restored normal vision to blind cataract victims. It was not easy to attract eye surgeons to help. To get things going, international organisations found it much easier to train doctors (and not eye surgeons) and even technicians to perform intracapsular cataract extraction without implant. This method, unfortunately, gave poor results. Half the patients remained blind after surgery as they did not have cataract glasses, and even if they had glasses, they suffered the agony of horrid optical disturbances described by the famous American ophthalmologist, Professor Alan Woods, in 1952.

In the late 1980s, several moves around the world were made to stop

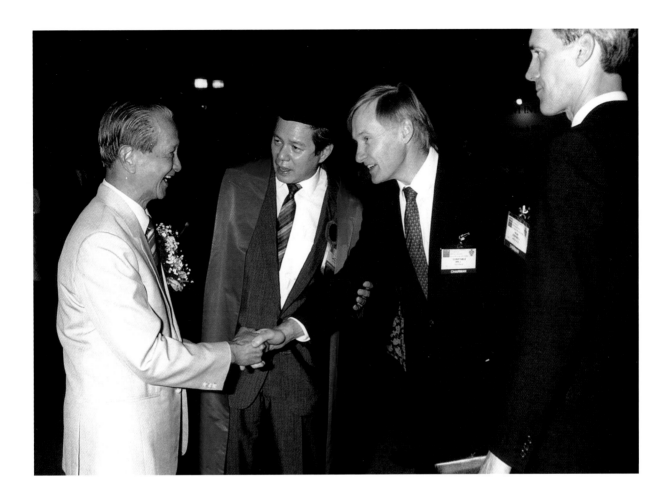

ICCE cataract surgery and to replace it with ECCE with PCI. A spectacular move was the establishment of the Tianjin Centre in the People's Republic of China, the first centre in the world dedicated to teaching microsurgery techniques and low-cost ECCE and PCI to eye surgeons. This centre was established in 1989 after three years of planning.

Asia's international standing in ophthalmology was sealed at the 26th International Congress of Ophthalmology (1990). Attracting over 8,000 ophthalmologists from around the world, the congress was a resounding success. Perhaps the most important achievement was that a thousand eye surgeons participated in the discussion on cataract blindness and the need to introduce modern techniques to benefit the rural areas

From left: President Wee Kim Wee, author, Professor Ian Constable and Professor Stephen Ryan at the 26th International Congress of Ophthalmology (1990)

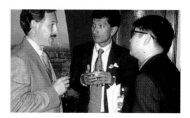

The 28th ICO, Amsterdam: In deep conversation are (from right) Dr Donald Tan, Deputy Medical Director, SNEC; Dr Vivian Balakrishnan, Medical Director, SNEC and Dr Olivier Schein, Consultant, Wilmer Eye Institute, Johns Hopkins University on the ongoing research collaborations between the two centres.

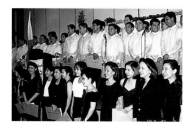

Looking resplendent in their national costumes are the graduates in Ophthalmology, who were amongst the participants of the 1997 Philippines Academy of Ophthalmology Annual Convention.

of developing countries. Recognizing this, Rolf Blach, Dean of the Institute of Ophthalmology, London, wrote:

> *"... no doubt that the energy, the enthusiasm and the imagination of one man (Arthur Lim) lifted the XXVI conference from yet another tired world jamboree to a mission to spread the word of the application of modern technological ophthalmology to the underprivileged masses of the world ..."*

The year 1990 also marked the inception of the Singapore National Eye Centre (SNEC). It is the designated national centre for clinical service, education and research in ophthalmology, centralizing ophthalmic specialist manpower, sophisticated facilities and equipment in one centre to deliver the highest standard of eye-care to patients in Singapore, Asia and beyond.

Spurred on by the spectacular success of the 1990 world congress, Asian eye surgeons introduced modern technology in the poor rural areas of Asia. Five centres in the People's Republic of China were established to train eye surgeons to perform low-cost quality ECCE and PCI, as well as to restore normal vision to the thousands blinded by cataract.

Unfortunately, some international organisations continued to be negative. The 1995 correspondence between a Director of the World Health Organisation, Bjorn Thylefors, and the author highlighted the resistance of international organisations to change from ICCE to ECCE with implant. Our differences, in my opinion, are essential for progress, as the world will not move forward if alternative approaches are not debated on openly and frankly. Hugh Taylor (1995) reported that:

> *"Although half the blindness worldwide is due to cataract, in most cases, blindness can be reversed by appropriate cataract surgery; 5 out of 6 people who are blind from cataract will die without having had cataract surgery."*

Taylor's gloomy report compels us to reflect on our failure in the battle against mass cataract blindness.

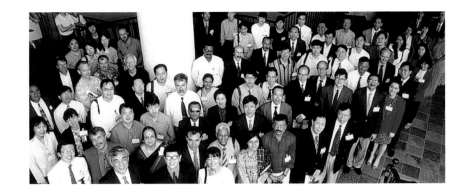

The Inaugural Scientific Meeting of the Asia Pacific Society of Cornea and Refractive Surgery held at Sentosa island and SNEC from March 27-30, 1997 attracted more than 300 ophthalmologists from 40 countries.

The establishment of WORLDCATS (now known as WORLDEYES or World Eye Surgeons Society) in 1994 was a swift response to the crisis of mass blindness. WORLDEYES today has the support of over 1,000 eye volunteers from 94 countries around the world. In our battle against mass blindness, let us always remember the words of Sir John Wilson:

> *"Only in statistics do people go blind by the millions. Each person goes blind by himself."*

Let us never forget the needs and the misery of every individual blind person. A poignant example is Ms Rokhaiya binte Shaikh Hussein who was registered blind for over 10 years, and had normal vision restored. Despite this, she had to learn to read all over again, letter by letter, since she had been trained to read in Braille. The path of a blind person is fraught with obstacles — in moving forwards, and in dealing with millions of blind people, it is essential that the individual blind person must never be forgotten.

I congratulate WHO and the NGOs for their recent change from ICCE to ECCE and PCI, for I know how difficult and painful it is for large organisations to change direction. Let us always remember that disagreements are a healthy stimulus for change and progress.

If we can overcome the resistance to change in this millennium,

The Day Light Dawned on Rokhai

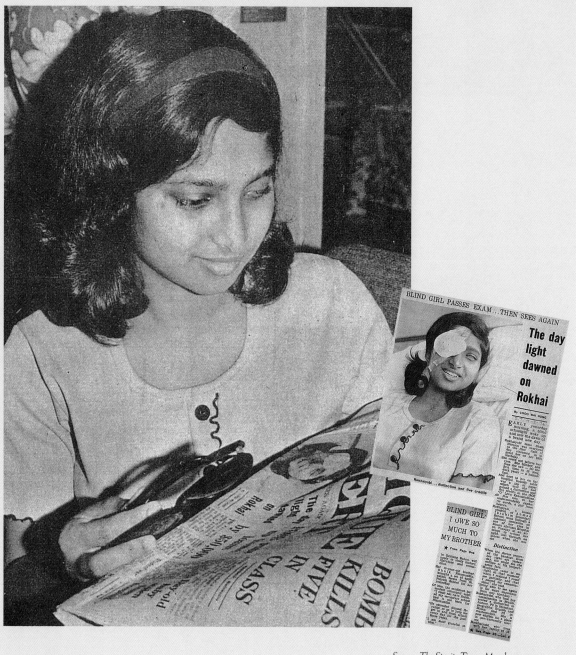

Source: *The Straits Times, March 11, 1976*

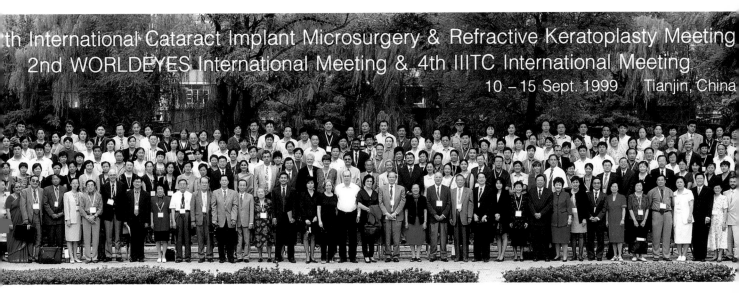

th International Cataract Implant Microsurgery & Refractive Keratoplasty Meeting
2nd WORLDEYES International Meeting & 4th IIITC International Meeting
10 – 15 Sept. 1999   Tianjin, China

we will usher in a glorious era, showering benefits on everyone in every country.

The various ophthalmic events that took place in September 1999, China, strengthened our faith in the power of international cooperation. In Beijing, the World Health Organisation convened the WHO/ Ministry of Health/International NGDO Third Coordination Meeting for the Prevention of Blindness. This was followed closely by the General Assembly of the International Agency for the Prevention of Blindness (IAPB). During this period, the newly established Beijing Medical University/Chinese University of Hong Kong Joint Eye Centre held a ground-breaking ceremony on 5 September 1999. The establishment of the eye centre was funded with a donation of US$2,000,000 by the Lam-Woo Foundation.

Many guests proceeded on to Tianjin to celebrate the 10th Anniversary of the International Intraocular Implant Training Centre (IIITC) and participated in their 4th international meeting held conjointly with the 12th ICIMRK and 2nd WORLDEYES International Meeting. This

The perfect finish to a prestigious gathering of leading ophthalmologists and administrators from around the world gathered in Tianjin at the 10th Anniversary of the International Intraocular Implant Training Centre (IIITC).

International Meetings in China

September 1999 in China would be memorable to many Chinese ophthalmologists from Tianjin and Beijing as they were hosts to 3 international ophthalmic conferences.

In Beijing, the World Health Organisation convened the WHO/Ministry of Health/International NGDO Third Coordination Meeting for the Prevention of Blindness. This was followed closely by the General Assembly of the International Agency for the Prevention of Blindness (IAPB). During this period, the newly established Beijing Medical University /Chinese University of Hong Kong Joint Eye Centre held a groundbreaking ceremony on 5 September 1999. The establishment of the eye centre was funded with a donation of US$2,000,000 by the Lam-Woo Foundation.

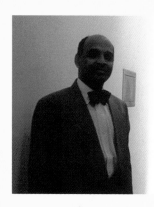
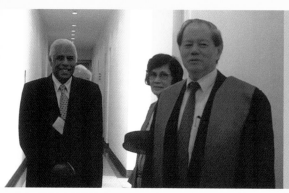

Dr Gullapalli Rao (Secretary-General, IAPB), Dr R Parajasegaram (Immediate Past-President, IAPB), Mrs A Lim and Prof Lim (Founder President, WORLDEYES)

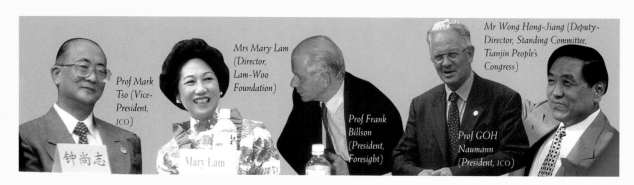

Prof Mark Tso (Vice-President, ICO)

Mrs Mary Lam (Director, Lam-Woo Foundation)

Prof Frank Billson (President, Foresight)

Mr Wong Hong-Jiang (Deputy-Director, Standing Committee, Tianjin People's Congress)

Prof GOH Naumann (President, ICO)

Many guests proceeded on to Tainjin to celebrate the 10th Anniversary of the International Intraocular Implant Training Centre Tianjin (IIITC) and participated in their 4th international meeting held conjointly with the 12th ICIMRK and 2nd WORLDEYES International Meeting.

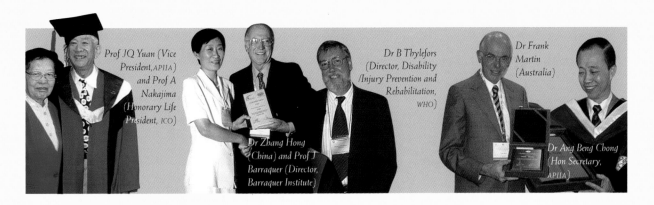

Prof JQ Yuan (Vice President, APIIA) and Prof A Nakajima (Honorary Life President, ICO)

Dr Zhang Hong (China) and Prof J Barraquer (Director, Barraquer Institute)

Dr B Thylefors (Director, Disability /Injury Prevention and Rehabilitation, WHO)

Dr Frank Martin (Australia)

Dr Ang Beng Chong (Hon Secretary, APIIA)

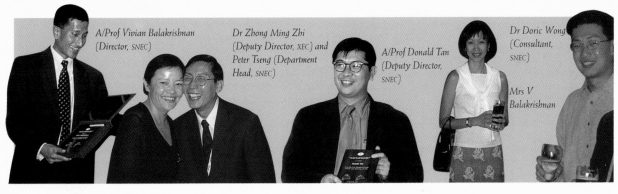

A/Prof Vivian Balakrishnan (Director, SNEC)

Dr Zhong Ming Zhi (Deputy Director, XEC) and Peter Tseng (Department Head, SNEC)

A/Prof Donald Tan (Deputy Director, SNEC)

Dr Doric Wong (Consultant, SNEC)

Mrs V Balakrishnan

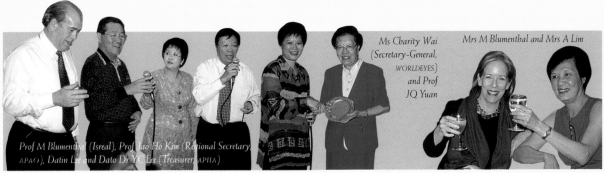

Ms Charity Wai (Secretary-General, WORLDEYES) and Prof JQ Yuan

Mrs M Blumenthal and Mrs A Lim

Prof M Blumenthal (Isreal), Prof Jao Ho Kim (Regional Secretary, APAO), Datin Lee and Dato Dr YC Lee (Treasurer, APIIA)

OPENING CEREMONY ADDRESS

Professor Arthur SM Lim

XXVIIIth International Congress of Ophthalmology, Amsterdam, 21-26 June 1998

What a great honour it is to speak on behalf of Asia to such a distinguished audience at this magnificent international meeting.

Let me begin by thanking the numerous leading ophthalmologists from Europe and America, such as August Deutman, who for many years, have helped Asia with repeated teaching visits, frequently at their own expense. Thank you.

The 20th Century brought sweeping revolutionary changes throughout Asia. In the early decades, Asia was poor and millions suffered the abuses of colonial rule and the horrors of war.

After the second world war, nationalism and independence was followed by rapid economic growth spreading throughout Asia.

And despite the current severe financial turmoil, Asia will emerge more united, more affluent, and more determined to succeed in the 21st Century. In addition, the people of Asia will demand quality healthcare.

Thus, Asia will see health expenditure exploding into billions of dollars per annum. These changes have already attracted numerous manufacturers, and eye surgeons from Europe and America to Asia.

In the 19th Century, Europe dominated the world. In the 20th Century, America emerged.

In the 21st century, we can expect Asia to compete for international leadership and Asia will continue to insist on fair and equitable Asian representation in international ophthalmic organizations.

As the world moves forward, eye surgeons will face numerous challenges:

- Information technology
- High technology
- Demand for quality
- Competition
- And increased costs.

We will also see extensive reforms in ophthalmology in every nation. But, let us remember that the interest of our patients must always be foremost.

Everyone can benefit if we can work together, respecting the cultures, the problems, the priorities and the needs of each nation.

Furthermore, information of the latest technology will spread to rural Asia and poor Asians blinded by cataract will demand normal vision with low-cost ECCE and implant.

International Organisations will be severely criticized in the 21st Century if they continue to perform another 10 million ICCEs.

For half will remain blind because they have no cataract glasses, and the other 5 million will be tormented by the horrid optical disturbance of cataract glasses so eloquently described in 1952 by the famous American ophthalmologist, the late Professor Alan Woods.

In the 21st Century, let us remember that if we are not open, the door to progress will be closed. I pray that quality care will be provided for all patients — especially to those who have little, in the 21st Century.

To the eye surgeons present, I would say:

"Let us work together for the benefit of mankind."

I appeal to the leading surgeons of the developed nations of Europe and America to continue to help your colleagues in the developing nations of Asia in order that quality care can be provided for all patients, especially those who have little, in the 21st century. ✢

prestigious gathering of ophthalmic luminaries signaled the beginning of a glorious era of international cooperation in ophthalmology. It is only when ophthalmologists work together in unity and with compassion that the citizens of the world can enjoy the wonders of modern eye-care.

The stage is set for the world to move forward so that every citizen in every nation can reap the benefits of modern ophthalmology. Singapore is also poised for major medical reforms so as to confront successfully the challenges of the 21st century. Let us, in the coming decade, work together, discuss major issues frankly and attempt to answer these challenges:

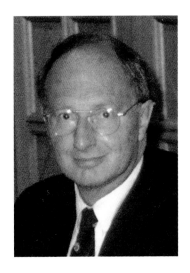

Prof August Deutman, President XXVIIIth ICO Congress in Amsterdam.

Where are we? What do we hope to achieve? Who should lead? WHO, NGOs? Private Organisations?

Should WHO be less centralized, with more representatives from developing countries?

Is IAPB too centralized? Are they achieving their objectives?

Will the prevention of blindness and ophthalmic development be more effective on a regional basis?

Is there adequate representation of developing nations in the International Council of Ophthalmology?

Are international congresses of ophthalmology too infrequent in developing nations?

Can governments continue to shut their eyes to the crisis of mass blindness?

Can governments ignore rising demand for quality eye-care?

What role should administrators, nutritionists and public health workers play in this millennium? What about eye surgeons?

More importantly, what is the role of eye surgeons? Will they not be key figures in the 21st century? As the incidence of major blinding

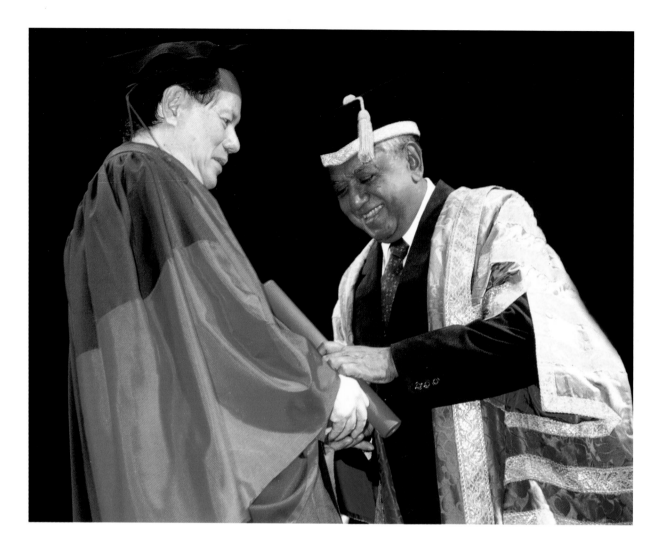

Professor Arthur Lim receiving the Honorary Degree of Doctor of Medicine from SR Nathan, President, Republic of Singapore, for his contribution to national and international ophthalmology (1999).

conditions such as cataract, glaucoma and diabetic retinopathy rapidly increases, will the world not need competent and dedicated eye surgeons?

How can we ensure quality eye-care for everyone, especially for those who are impoverished and have little hope in life? How will the massive changes of the 21st century affect eye-care? Will eye surgeons reform and respond urgently to ride the tide? Will ophthalmology drift if no clear direction is established?

Let more active practising eye surgeons — especially those from developing nations — help us move forward in the 21st century. We must remember the famous words of Theodore Roosevelt who spoke about the man in the arena:

> *"It is not the critic who counts; not the man who points out how the strong man stumbles, or where the doer of deeds could have done them better. The credit belongs to the man who is actually in the arena, whose face is marred by dust and sweat and blood; who strives valiantly..."*

There are no easy answers to the challenges and controversies of this millennium. I believe that the 21st century will be a glorious era when the wonders of modern eye-care will spread to the peoples of the world. Let us remember the world will not judge us by what we say, but by what we do. Let us act and move forward! ✳

Chapter 2

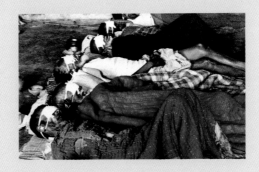

"I Want to See"

Chapter 2

"I Want to See"

"I want to see" will be the cry of 10 million cataract victims after intracapsular cataract extraction (ICCE).

International organisations will be severely criticized if they continue to recommend another 10 million ICCEs for blind cataract victims. Five million will remain blind because they have no cataract glasses; and because of cataract glasses, the other 5 million usually suffer the agony of optical disturbances so eloquently described in the 1952 American Journal of Ophthalmology editorial by the eminent American professor, Alan Woods[1], himself a victim of cataract glasses after ICCE.

Eye surgeons who performed cataract surgery without implants 30 years ago would frequently have to listen to intensely unhappy patients, who despite successful ICCE, would prefer to remain blind without cataract glasses, as they could not tolerate cataract glasses.

In 1990, Sommer[2] reported that, "At least half of the people who have undergone allegedly successful surgery are blind, because they do not have aphakic glasses."

The ophthalmic aberrations, the distortion of images, the enlarged images, the problem of judging distances, the limited field of vision, and the jack-in-the-box phenomenon become terrifying

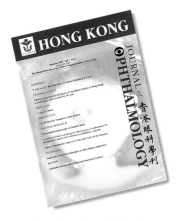

Editorial by author published in the Hong Kong Journal of Ophthalmology, October 1997, Volume 1, No. 3

for the patients, especially when their cataract spectacles are ill fitting and of poor quality. Walking and physical activity requiring vision become difficult, even dangerous. These are the optical horrors of the 50% of patients termed successes, as described in Sommer's report.

Why are the international organisations still recommending ICCE? Why is an obsolete operation that is no longer used in the West and in the major cities of Asia still recommended for the poor, rural blind cataract victims of the People's Republic of China? What is the justification?

I will write frankly, because if we are not open to alternative views, we will close the door to truth and lock out solutions to cataract blindness in the 21st century.

It has been estimated that blindness from cataract in the world may increase from 20 to 40 million in 10 years. In addition, in 1995, Taylor[3] stunned us with the analysis that only 1 of 6 blind cataract victims underwent surgery and the other 5 died without surgery.

Why have we failed when normal vision can be restored to all patients today at low costs? Why should this happen when, for 20 years, the World Health Organisation (WHO), the International Agency for the Prevention of Blindness, and many other international organisations have been spending millions of dollars every year to combat world blindness?

We know that one reason is the increased number of patients who suffer blindness from cataract because people now live longer. Another reason is the resistance of international organisations to new approaches.

For example, these organisations have been indifferent to the successful and exciting new approach to teach extracapsular cata-

Why have we failed when normal vision can be restored to all patients today at low costs? Why should this happen when, for 20 years, the World Health Organisation (WHO), the International Agency for the Prevention of Blindness, and many other international organisations have been spending millions of dollars every year to combat world blindness?

ract extraction (ECCE) and posterior chamber intraocular lens implantation (PCIOL) by setting up training centres in developing nations.

In 1989, the Tianjin International Intraocular Implant Training Centre[4] was formed, and by 1998, it will have trained 2,000 ophthalmologists. The Centre is founded on one basic principle: "Each time you perform a cataract surgery, you restore sight to one man. But if you teach quality cataract surgery to your fellow eye surgeons, you will restore sight to millions."

By working with other centres, the Tianjin Centre hopes to restore normal vision to 1 million people in 5 years. With the establishment of more training centres, 10,000 eye surgeons can be trained in 5 years. If each performs 200 cataract operations a year, this would mean 2 million cataract operations performed each year. The Tianjin Centre has succeeded, let the world follow.

Success in controlling cataract blindness in the People's Republic of China will be historic, as the world has failed after 20 years.

I appeal to the eye surgeons of Asia to teach their Asian colleagues low-cost ECCE with lens implantation. For what greater value have eye surgeons to their profession than to help restore vision to the blind? I also appeal to all eye surgeons of the world to work with Asian eye surgeons so that we can succeed rapidly.

World Bank

I appeal to the WHO and to international non-governmental organisations (NGOs) to follow the historic programme that the World Bank[5] has planned for India. If we can work together, we can control this major world surgical problem within 10 years in the People's Republic of China.

In 1989, the Tianjin International Intraocular Implant Trining Centre was formed, and by 1998, it will have trained 2,000 ophthalmologists. The Centre is founded on one basic principle: "Each time you perform a cataract surgery, you restore sight to one man. But if you teach quality cataract surgery to your fellow eye surgeons, you will restore sight to millions."

On June 11, 1996, the World Bank explained its outstanding and practical approach to the problem of cataract blindness in India. The plan is to restore vision to 11 million cataract victims in the country in 5 years, with a loan of more than $100 million to the Indian government.

The key steps introduced in India are similar to those used in Tianjin. The World Bank programme includes the following:

- Promoting a rapid change to ECCE.
- Training medical students in 7 medical colleges to perform ECCE, as well as training more than 1,500 government surgeons.
- Encouraging private physicians to work together with NGOs and governments to provide quality surgery to the poor.
- Building and equipping facilities for ECCE.

Few people expected the World Bank to initiate such a wonderful programme in India. It would be useful for China to study the World Bank's programme and to consider adopting what is appropriate. Let me emphasize: "When the human misery of millions of blind cataract victims continues to increase in the poor areas of our world, at a time when medical advances can restore normal vision to them at low costs, we will press for change, for action."[6]

The 21st Century

It is sad how opposition to major changes in surgery can delay progress. It is human nature to resist change and this has become the major obstacle to success in the control of mass cataract blindness.

Fortunately, the tide is changing.

In the 21st century, ECCE with PCI will be universally accepted. This is because the governments and leaders of Asia cannot close their eyes to the millions blind from cataract, any more than they can close their eyes to the needs of housing, education, food, transportation, and basic medical care.

In addition, phacoemulsification and other methods of small incision cataract surgery with foldable implants, with their advantage of rapid rehabilitation, have already spread to all Asian cities and the more developed areas of Asia. Although phacoemulsification remains controversial in eye camps, it has been recently successfully performed in India. It is wrong not to move forward in the twenty-first century.

China's success will be historic, and Tianjin will be a model for all other developing countries to follow in the 21st century. There is a saying: "It is easier to stop an invading army than to stop a right idea at the right time."[7]

The solution to mass cataract blindness in the People's Republic of China is complex and difficult, requiring us to work together for success. I appeal for unity.

I appeal for ECCE and implants for all cataract victims as we must respond to their cry, "I want to see!" ✳

In the 21st century, ECCE with PCI will be universally accepted. This is because the governments and leaders of Asia cannot close their eyes to the millions blind from cataract, any more than they can close their eyes to the needs of housing, education, food, transportation, and basic medical care.

Editorial by author published in the Hong Kong Journal of Ophthalmology, October 1997, Volume 1, No. 3

Chapter 3

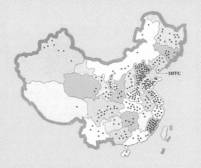

Tianjin Centre
A Model for the World
to Follow

The Tianjin Centre has trained 2,250 eye surgeons and has restored normal vision to 120,000 blind cataract victims with low-cost extracapsular cataract extraction and lens implantation. A trail-blazer in ophthalmic training and services, it has plans to restore vision to 1,000,000 blind victims in conjunction with other centres in the People's Republic of China. It has also paved the way for the establishment of like centres around the world.

Contributed by

Yuan Jia-Qin, Honorary Director,

International Intraocular Implant Training Centre, Tianjin, China

Chapter 3

Tianjin Centre:
A Model for the World
to Follow

This is a wonderful 20th century model of success in restoring normal vision to patients blinded by cataract. It is the first centre in the world to be built exclusively for ECCE and implant surgery, and operates with the primary objective that "If you give a man a fish, you can feed him for a day. But if you teach him how to fish, he can feed himself for a lifetime." After 10 years, the Tianjin Centre has become a resounding success in teaching 2,250 eye surgeons and in restoring, through modern low-cost cataract surgery, normal vision to 120,000 blind cataract victims. Together with other centres in China, it plans to achieve the target of 1,000,000 operations.

The International Intraocular Implant Training Centre (IIITC) in Tianjin, China.

In this decade, surgical management of cataract in developing nations will continue to be controversial. It is a problem of quality versus quantity — a problem of how to deal with mass cataract blindness with limited resources.

Several essential questions have to be answered:

(1)   Is implant surgery for mass cataract blindness appropriate?

(2) If it is, which is the recommended method?

(3) What are the major problems with ECCE and PCI?

(4) Can these problems be overcome?

(5) How do we train ophthalmologists to perform ECCE with PCI?

How do we train ophthalmologists? This is most important.

Training must emphasize cost-effective methods. The technique must be simple and inexpensive but effective — the Simcoe or McIntyre cannula is appropriate. It is wrong to introduce phacoemulsification, and automated infusion/aspiration systems are unnecessary. It is important to emphasize that a good microscope with good co-axial light is essential — the simpler models such as Zeiss I or Topcon 80 are adequate. Quality implants must be used, as badly manufactured implants can lead to blinding complications. Ensuring sterile methods and the use of sterile buffered salt solution and viscoelastic material must be taught and their value explained.

Basic Techniques of Microsurgery

"An ophthalmologist who is comfortable with the operating microscope will find learning ECCE and PCI easy; but for one who is not familiar with it, unnecessary complications will be common". Training of ECCE and PCI implant surgeons must be based on this essential principle.

The first essential is learning basic microsurgical techniques. In developed countries, young ophthalmologists begin their training with the operating microscope so this is not a problem. However, in developing countries, the microscope is not usually used in training or in practice (by the majority of surgeons when performing cataract extraction).

The training of a surgeon who has performed thousands of cataracts with an operating loupe is a major obstacle. This is because of a number

Training must emphasize cost-effective methods.

An ophthalmologist who is comfortable with the operating microscope will find learning ECCE and PCI easy... .

of inherent difficulties in microsurgery for experienced surgeons. In contrast to the "mobility" when using the loupe, they are confined to a "static" position with the microscope. In addition, the high magnification limits the field of vision and the surgeon becomes a "prisoner" within a narrow field of vision.

In the early 1970s, most surgeons in South-East Asia and many developed countries did not use operating microscopes. The problem was overcome when hundreds of ophthalmologists attended numerous courses organised in Singapore and elsewhere in Asia. Thus, training for ECCE and PCI in South-East Asia was easy. But most ophthalmologists in India and the People's Republic of China have not been trained to use the operating microscope. This is still the main obstacle in these countries.

At present, less than 30% of eye surgeons in the developing nations use the operating microscope. This was the situation 30 years ago, in Europe, America and Australia. Because of this, numerous microsurgical teaching courses were held throughout the world. In South-East Asia alone, hundreds of ophthalmologists were trained to use the operating microscope. Numerous courses were conducted by Ang Beng Chong, Singapore; Joaquin Barraquer, Spain; Ian Constable, Australia; August Deutman, Netherlands; Dick Galbraith, Australia; Arthur Lim, Singapore; Saiichi Mishima, Japan; Tom Moore, USA and Noel Rice, London. As a result, ophthalmic microsurgery is a routine in South-East Asia and in the developing nations.

With rapid communication and expanding economies, I predict that ophthalmic microsurgical techniques will be firmly established throughout Asia in 10 years, given support from the developed nations and microsurgical teachers of Asia. It is clear that the introduction of microsurgery will reduce blindness, not only from cataract, but also from corneal disease, glaucoma, severe trauma and vitreoretinal diseases.

ECCE and implantation

The best training is the traditional Resident's training programme or alternatively, the establishment of a national implant training centre. Unfortunately, for the vast majority of surgeons, especially those already in practice, this is not practical. Thus, short courses or short attachments, training in a laboratory, video-tape teaching, books and journals are alternative methods of training.

Tianjin project

Because of the advantages of formal training, it was decided after much discussion with the ophthalmologists and administrators of the Tianjin Province, People's Republic of China, that an international training centre be established in Tianjin. This centre would serve as a base hospital for training and supervision of work done in the county (regional) hospitals. Through the regional hospitals, implant surgery can be extended to villages and small towns. Thus a three-tier system has been created.

A three-tier system has been created.

(1) The International Intraocular Implant Training Centre affiliated to the Tianjin Medical University.

(2) A county hospital (the Jixian County Hospital and more recently, the Baodi County Hospital and Jinghai County Hospital).

(3) A village hospital.

The regional hospital, being service-orientated, pre-empts the over loading of the teaching hospital and the training centre in service commitments.

Important ingredients for success include a dedicated ophthalmic leader — this was found in Professor Yuan Jia-Qin, the Professor of Ophthalmology, Tianjin Medical College and a dedicated and outstanding leader of ophthalmology. Furthermore, support from the university and the government is crucial for success. The project in Tianjin is fortunate to have the personal support of Professor Wu Hsein-chung, the President of the Tianjin Medical College, and Mr Wang En-Lui, the ex-mayor of Tianjin, who underwent implant surgery successfully in 1986.

Other important factors include international ophthalmologists who helped to ensure international standard. The ophthalmologists include Professors Kensaku Miyake, Akira Momose and Saiichi Mishima of Japan; Robert Sinskey, Jack Dodick, Stephen Obstbaum and Maurice Luntz of USA; Douglas Coster, Frank Billson and Ian Constable of Australia; BC Ang and Arthur Lim of Singapore; and Noel Rice, Emanuel Rosen and Bo Philipson of Europe.

The Tianjin International Intraocular Implant Training Centre was opened on 29 September 1989.

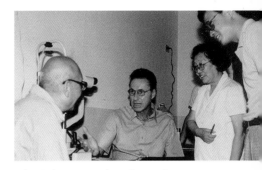

Robert Sinskey, an outstanding and renowned implant surgeon from California, USA, regularly demonstrates the latest surgical techniques at the Tianjin centre.

The Tianjin Centre is indebted to the following ophthalmologists: Professors Kensaku Miyake, Akira Momose and Saiichi Mishima; Robert Sinskey, Jack Dodick, Stephen Obstbaum and Maurice Luntz; Douglas Coster, Frank Billson and Ian Constable; BC Ang and Arthur Lim; Noel Rice, Emanuel Rosen and Bo Philipson

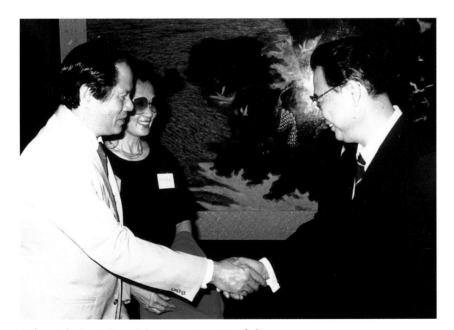

Professor Arthur Lim met Premier Li Peng in 1988 in recognition for his contribution to ophthalmology in the People's Republic of China.

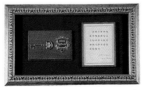

Tianjin honorary citizenship and golden key to Tianjin city awarded to Professor Arthur Lim in May, 1991.

Tianjin, a major city in the northern part of the People's Republic of China, is an hour's drive from Beijing and serves as the capital city to a province of 10 million. It is relatively prosperous and organised, and is a good choice as it has the support of the provincial government, the University and most importantly, a dedicated professor of ophthalmology — Professor Yuan Jia-Qin — supported by her team of ophthalmologists.

Professor Yuan Jia-Qin has a special message which reads "The Centre is determined to do its utmost in carrying out faithfully the purpose of its establishment to introduce the most advanced techniques to my country, to promote the spirit of friendship and international cooperation, to train highly-skilled ophthalmologists, to restore eyesight to those who have lost it and to bring happiness to people."

An important step in the project was the organisation of a basic microsurgical teaching course in 1988. This was done by Noel Rice, Frank Billson, BC Ang and Arthur Lim in Tianjin where 40 ophthalmologists from various parts of China attended. After this course, several other courses have been organised in different parts of China. Thus the programme is not only limited to the province of Tianjin with a population of 10 million, but may influence implant surgery throughout the whole of China.

This centre has progressed well since it was established in 1989. Over the past ten years, the centre has successfully performed 40,000 implant operations. Another 50,000 implant operations were performed with other related centres in the country. More than 2,500 ophthalmologists from all parts of China have been trained at the IIITC. The centre has also sent working groups to 93 hospitals in the different parts of rural China to help them train and perform implant surgery.

Five ophthalmologists have been honoured by the provincial government for their contributions to the country. Professor Yuan

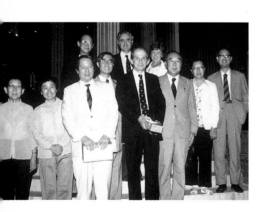

Prof Arthur Lim, Prof Frank Billson and Dr Noel Rice were the Course Directors of the basic microsurgical teaching course at the IIITC in 1988.

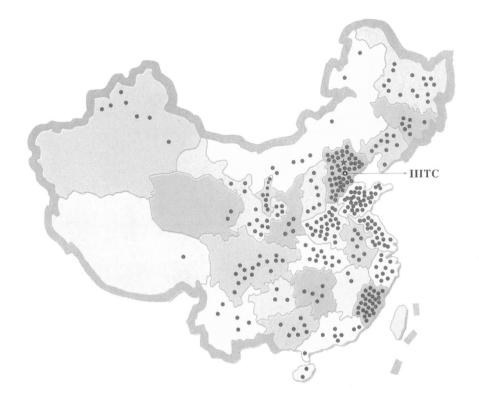

IIITC

The red dots are areas from where ophthalmologists were taught ECCE and PCI.

Jia-Qin, Director of the IIITC, was recently presented an award by the State for her outstanding work in the control of cataract blindness.

The IIITC has restored normal vision to 120,000 blind cataract victims. With the co-operation of the Xiamen and Jinan Centres, I believe that 1,000,000 implant operations can be achieved in the near future.

Tianjin's project can be a model upon which similar systems can be established throughout the world — with variations to suit local requirements.

There is no short cut to acquiring skills. Ophthalmologists without the necessary experience must be adequately trained and supervised before being allowed to perform implant surgery. They must not perform implant surgery unsupervised before they have had sufficient experience to minimise risk to the patient's vision.

Conclusion

The training of ophthalmologists in microsurgery, ECCE and PCI may be painfully slow. In many communities, a system similar to the Tianjin Project may be appropriate. If we act now, thousands of cataract victims throughout the developing world will benefit from the wonderful progress of cataract technology. ✳

Tianjin: Chronicling 10 Years of Spectacular Success

"On September 29, 1989, the sun was beaming and the coloured flags were fluttering gaily in the wind. The distinctive building of the Tianjin Centre, striking an ebullient pose by the Jinyi Lake, attracted both Chinese and foreign guests."

Professor Yuan Jia-Qin, Spreading Light Across China

In September 1989, when the Tianjin Centre was opened, I quietly wondered with concern whether it would be easier for an elephant to scale the Great Wall of China than for Professor Yuan Jia-Qin to establish a successful leading cataract centre, influencing the world to restore normal vision to thousands of cataract victims. My suspicions were unfounded. Since then, the Centre has come a long way in treating numerous cases of cataract blindness, training a large number of ophthalmologists in low-cost ECCE and PCI, and establishing strong inter-national links all over the world. Professor Yuan Jia-Qin, I sincerely salute you.

The Tianjin Centre would have been a quixotic project without the firm support of the State Council and the Tianjin Municipal Government, as well as generous donations from Prof Kensaku Miyake and Prof Akira Momose of Japan and other foreign well-wishers. I gave my humble contribution as well.

Under the beneficent steward-ship of Prof Yuan, the level of intel-lectual exchange between the Tianjin Centre and other parts of China and the world has increased. Over the years, well-known international experts from Singapore, the United States, the United Kingdom, Belgium, India, Hong Kong, Australia, Canada, Sweden, Spain and Japan have been invited to conduct lectures or demonstrate live surgery, and some have even visited more than once. These foreign specialists, as well as those from other parts of China, introduced advanced techniques and the latest equipment to the local doctors. In addition, the Tianjin Centre has successfully organised three international meetings in 1991,

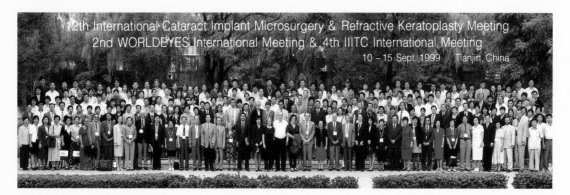

Participants at a recent international meeting in Tianjin in September 1999.

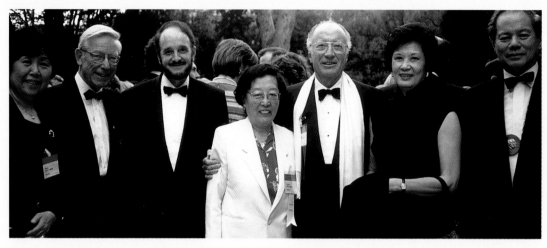

Prof Yuan Jia-Qin and Prof Sun Hui-Min of IIITC attending the 50th anniversary of the Barraquer Instituto in Spain. (L-R) Prof Sun, Dr R Drews (USA), Prof J Murube (Spain), Prof Yuan, Prof J Barraquer (Spain), Mrs A Lim and Prof A Lim (Singapore).

1993 and 1996, attracting a total of 400 experts from more than 40 countries. Then in September 1999, the Centre ran the 12th ICIMRK, 2nd WORLDEYES and 4th IIITC international meetings in conjunction with its 10th anniversary celebrations. From its humble origins as a training ground for eye surgeons in cataract implant surgery, the Tianjin Centre has flourished into a global model for surgical skills development. This has broad ramifications for like centres around the world.

"They (international friends) are what encourage me forward. Their one word or one letter greatly inspires me. We could not have had today's success without their generosity and kindness. My heart cannot help leaping and rejoicing, "Long live international friendship!"

Professor Yuan Jia-Qin, Spreading Light Across China

Of the visiting international experts, world-leading ophthalmologist Prof Joaquin Barraquer of Spain was of great inspiration to the leaders of the Tianjin Centre. In 1997, Prof Yuan and Prof Sun Hui-Min of the Tianjin Centre were invited to Barcelona for the 50th anniversary celebrations of the Barraquer Institute. Their resources included inventions, scientific books and pathological specimens, collected by the Barraquer family through the years. The buildings, structure and overall organisation of the Institute

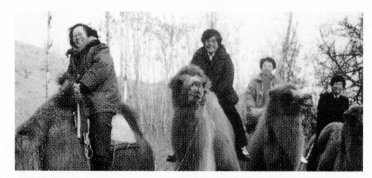

Prof Yuan leading an operation team to Ningxia Autonomous Region to help develop cataract implant surgery.

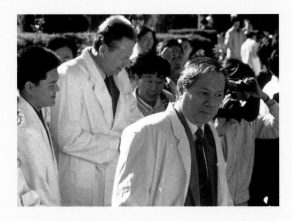

Prof Arthur Lim and Prof Robert Sinskey assisting at the free eye screening campaign.

and the hospital, especially the unique design of the operating theatre, left a deep impression on Prof Yuan and Prof Sun.

Another area of strong focus for the Tianjin Centre is the training of Chinese and foreign doctors. Besides having postgraduate students from the Tianjin Medical University, the Centre has accepted some 160 ophthalmologists from many parts of China, including Tibet and Taiwan, for intensive training attachments of three to six months. These ophthalmologists worked as assistant residents, attending outpatient clinics, looking after patients in the wards, assisting in surgery and performing wet lab surgeries. Dr Mau Imo of Samoa was the first foreign ophthalmologist to undergo a 10-month attachment programme in the Centre, and ophthalmologists from other developing countries expressed interest to study there.

At the same time, ophthalmologists representing the Centre visited other parts of China to help local hospitals develop implant surgery and treat complicated eye diseases, and to conduct training courses.

Next, 17 of the best doctors and nurses from the Centre were posted, one after another, to Singapore, Japan, the United States, Belgium, Spain and Russia for further studies or international conferences. These international meetings and opportunities not only enriched the experiences of the medical professionals, but also strengthened the Centre's friendly ties with foreign ophthalmologists.

The Tianjin Centre has entrenched itself in research as well. The clinical research carried out probes the experience of implant surgery, including the application of different types of IOL, the various methods and complications of IOL implant surgery,

secondary implantation, and implant surgery in children. As for basic and applied research, the focus is on the mechanism of opacity of posterior capsule of lens and the surface modification of IOLs. To date, the Centre has obtained some preliminary results in its research.

On September 1995, a grand celebration of the 6th anniversary of IIITC was held in Tianjin. In conjunction with the celebration, a massive screening project was carried out with WORLDEYES. Both Prof Robert Sinskey and I were involved.

"That night, all of us could not suppress our excitement as we pored over the plans for the centre's future. Professor Arthur Lim spoke glowingly of the prospects of IIITC, and thought that it had, right from the beginning, the potential to develop into an Eye Centre."

Professor Yuan Jia-Qin,
Spreading Light Across China

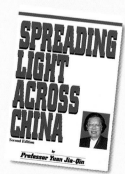

China honours Singaporean eye surgeon with top award

Recognition for helping to fight mass cataract blindness

By Mary Kwang
China Correspondent

BEIJING — Singaporean eye surgeon Professor Arthur Lim has won an international science and technology cooperation award from the Chinese government for helping to fight mass cataract blindness in that country.

The honour was given to Prof Lim by the State Science and Technology Commission (SSTC) for his contributions to ophthalmology technology. It was conferred alongside the country's most authoritative science and technology awards to local scientists.

A presentation ceremony was held at the Great Hall of the People on Friday for the scientists, officiated by President Jiang Zemin and attended by Premier Li Peng and Vice-Premiers Zhu Rongji and Li Lanqing.

Prof Lim, 63, who is the medical director of the Singapore National Eye Centre (SNEC), is one of two foreigners to win the honour this year.

The other winner is Mr Jean Pierre Lebrun of France for advancing Sino-European cooperation in the information field.

In a telephone interview, Prof Lim, who is in Singapore, said: "It's nice when Singapore, a small country, can work with a big country."

Giving credit to the people who work with him, he said: "It's teamwork. There are more than 10 eye doctors and administrative staff involved in the work."

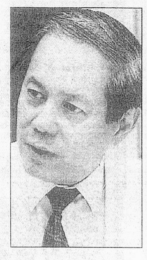

Other awards

Prof Lim (left) has received other honours from China:

■ Last year, he was given the Friendship Award by the Fujian government for his help in setting up the Xiamen Eye Centre.

■ He has also been made an honorary citizen of Tianjin.

The award is only the latest honour heaped by China on Prof Lim, who has carried out ophthalmology work in that country for 12 years, including leading teams of eye surgeons to hold surgery demonstrations and setting up eye centres.

China has millions of cataract victims, but there are not enough trained ophthalmologists to perform cataract implant surgery.

Last year, Prof Lim was given the Friendship Award by the Fujian government for his help in setting up the Xiamen Eye Centre. He has also been made an honorary citizen of Tianjin.

The SNEC coordinates and liaises with eye centres in China that provide training in surgery to local ophthalmologists. It also helps in raising funds for such centres. Till date, Singapore has helped set up five eye centres in China.

Prof Lim, who founded the World Cataract Surgeons Society and has support from the World Bank, does similar work in India, Vietnam and Myanmar.

He is also looking into opening eye centres in Bangladesh.

Complimenting the Chinese for being good surgeons and quick learners, he remarked: "I think this has to do with the Chinese using chopsticks.

"That helps them control well the small muscles in the hand. The instruments for the eye are held like chopsticks."

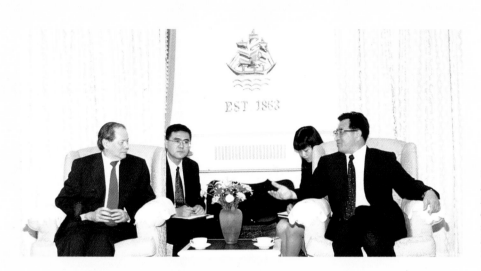

SNEC's Founding Medical Director, Prof Arthur Lim, exchanging views with Mr Li Sheng Lin, mayor of Tianjin.

We were not to be let down: the subsequent year saw funds and support pouring in from various quarters for the extension of phase II.

Happiness seldom comes in pairs. But when we gathered in Tianjin for its 10th anniversary in 1999, it was a cause for double celebration as the phase II extension had also been successfully completed. Our dream to make the Tianjin Eye Centre a reality had come true. It was indeed a timely occasion as we prepared the Centre, now a huge building with an area of 5,000m², to scale even greater heights in anticipation of the challenges of the 21st century.

This chapter is a tribute to all our supporters who have successfully led the Tianjin Centre to achieve great advances in medical treatment, training, scientific research and rural work. More than 2,250 doctors from all over the country have passed through the training doors of the Centre, and the previously unknown technique of IOL implantation has become popularised in the county hospitals. It is also heartening to know that the Centre has made impressive progress in conducting 120,000 cases of implant surgery to restore normal vision to blind cataract victims. In recognition of its tireless efforts in the prevention and treatment of blindness over the years, the Centre received 25 awards from international organisations, five from the Chinese Central Government and 23 from the Tianjin Municipality. Indeed, the Tianjin Eye Centre has become a successful model for teaching doctors to perform low-cost operations in developing countries. It is now poised to welcome fellow colleagues from all over the world and to provide quality services to patients in the 21st century. The soaring lyrics of "The Song of the Implant Training Centre" best capture its vision for the millennium:

"Oh, the Implant Training Centre
- symbol of mankind's cause bright.
... ...
The centre's fighters
cherish the lofty virtue
of overcoming difficulty and danger
with tenacity.
The world embraces us
and we march towards the world.
Let the globe be full of hope
and songs gay." ✢

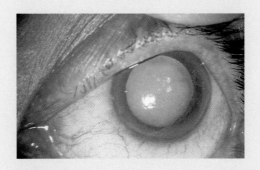

First Susruta Memorial Lecture
Increasing Importance of Eye Surgeons in Mass Cataract Blindness — a Megatrend

"The world needs competent eye surgeons to counter the rise of blinding conditions such as cataract, glaucoma and diabetic retinopathy."

Chapter 4

First Susruta Memorial Lecture: Increasing Importance of Eye Surgeons in Mass Cataract Blindness — a Megatrend

Bangladesh is one of the poorest countries in the world with hundreds of thousands of blind cataract victims. When the Susruta Lecture was established in 1993, the author was invited to deliver the first Susruta Lecture. His hour-long lecture emphasized the need for eye surgeons to participate more actively in combating mass cataract blindness. In 1994, the author founded the World Cataract Surgeons Society, which sought to stimulate the interest of eye surgeons worldwide to help relieve the misery of millions blind from cataract.

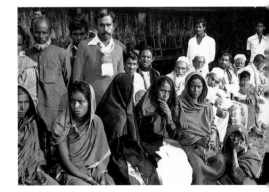

Crowd waiting

Introduction

The major causes of mass blindness have shifted from infection and malnutrition to cataract. By the 1970s, cataract accounted for 50% of mass blindness. As lifespan increases in many communities, cataract accounts for up to 80% of mass blindness today. Correspondingly, eye surgeons have become essential in the control of mass blindness.

Adapted from The First Susruta Memorial Lecture, 14th APAO Congress, January 1993.

Susruta

The story of cataract surgery is full of interest. Susruta, a native of ancient Bangladesh, was an ophthalmologist in about 1000 BC. He was known as the originator of cataract surgery. He practised cataract surgery by couching even before the Egyptians, Arabs, Greeks and Romans.

He was not only the greatest exponent of treating cataract with couching, but he also expounded that the foundation of surgery was based on anatomical dissections. He described with surprising accuracy the anatomy, physiology and pathology of the eye.

It would be interesting, were Susruta alive today, to know how he would approach today's problems of mass cataract blindness and cataract surgery.

The earliest written reference is found in the Sanskrit manuscripts, "Susruta Samhita" and "Uttara Tantra", dating from 5th century BC. He taught that the foundation of surgery was the anatomy; he classified ocular diseases systematically on a topographical basis and enumerated them in 76 varieties; he introduced antisepsis in surgery; he performed ingenious dissection; he constructed and

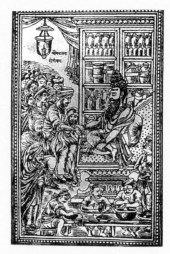

An Indian print of the 18th century showing Susruta teaching medicine.

modeled more than 100 surgical instruments in which some have no alternatives even today. Susruta was a man of great scientific acumen.

In the wealth of his teaching, he described several different varieties of cataract, giving an admirable account of the technique of its treatment by couching.

He used to fumigate his operating room with sulfur fumes and incense. Sulfur dioxide gas is a well known antiseptic and detergent, and incense fumes contain essential oils which also have antiseptic properties. Before proceeding with an operation, he used to take a bath and change his clothes, cut his nails as well as have his long hair tied in a knot on top of his head. Susruta definitely knew that preoperative cleanliness adopted by him would minimise postoperative complications.

Susruta, a genius and an outstanding ophthalmologist of ancient Bangladesh, not only contributed much to ophthalmology but also to medical science. ✢

With this worldwide trend, there is now a unique opportunity for eye surgeons to contribute their skills to help their fellowmen.

Current Situation of Mass Cataract Blindness

Let us review the problem of mass cataract blindness. Mass blindness will double in 10 years because blindness from cataract will increase with increased life expectancy. Cataract is a massive problem in Asia, accounting for more than 50% of blindness in the developing countries.

The backlog of unoperated patients is estimated to be over 10 million and this has caused major socio-economic problems.

Implant Surgery in Rural Areas of Developing Countries

It is my belief that, with time, demand for implant surgery will spread rapidly to every major hospital throughout Asia. It will also spread to the rural areas throughout Asia, although this may take one decade.

Numerous questions relating to the value of lens implantation for the rural population of the developing countries remain unanswered. These include: are there more complications with extracapsular cataract extraction (ECCE) and posterior chamber lens implantation (PCI) compared with intracapsular cataract extraction (ICCE) and anterior chamber lens implantation? Should ICCE and anterior chamber lens implants be used instead? Is it inappropriate for patients in the rural areas to have lens implantation — what is the risk-benefit ratio? Is the cost of ECCE and PCI significantly higher? Will implantation aggravate the backlog of cataract blindness as fewer patients can be operated on? These important questions are likely to remain unanswered.

I believe that the need to develop implant surgery in developing countries is so compelling, it would be wrong to delay action until statistics become available. It would be wrong not to move forward. Although lens implantation in the rural areas of the developing countries will increase costs — which include the cost of trained manpower, the cost of implant, the cost of sterile-buffered solution, the cost of operating microscope and the cost of viscoelastic material — it is clear that the demand for implants will grow in the cities. In the rural communities, its use will vary and in some areas, remain controversial. The main concern is the fear of complications and the lack of manpower and organisation besides the increased cost.

I believe that the need to develop implant surgery in developing countries is so compelling, it would be wrong to delay action... .

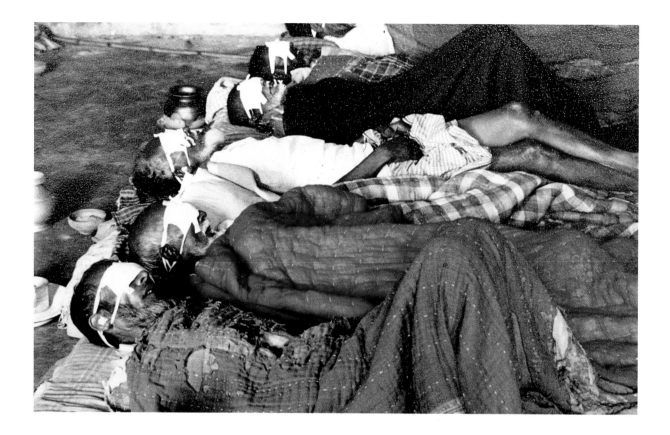

Cataract eye camps are temporary, with numerous problems and complications.
The trend is to develop static cataract centres

However, one strong reason in support of implantation is that the "normal" vision patients attain following successful lens implantation is such that it encourages other cataract victims from the villages to seek cataract surgery. This is a strong motivation for the neglected village cataract victims to seek implant surgery. The need for gongs, banners and campaigns to encourage villagers to come forward for surgery may then be unnecessary.

Increasing Importance of Eye Surgeons — a Megatrend

Besides cataract, glaucoma continues to be an important problem and in some communities, blindness from diabetic retinopathy and severe eye injury from industrial and traffic accidents have increased. All these conditions require eye surgery.

Thylefors and others have repeatedly stated that although the problem of mass cataract is well known, organisations have failed to translate this into action. There are many reasons for this. One of which is the lack of response and commitment of eye surgeons. Let us deliberate on the possible reasons why the responses of eye surgeons have not been good.

Prevention of blindness has, for decades, been the role of nutritionists and public health workers combined with lay volunteers. The surgeon's role has been nominal. Furthermore, there have been little or no incentives to attract eye surgeons to volunteer. Why should an eye surgeon leave the comfort of his city practice to work in the rural areas where there are no incentives and recognition? This must be changed.

As the increasing importance of eye surgeons is now clear, we need to create incentives to attract them.

In the late 1990s, the megatrend will be for eye surgeons worldwide to help control mass cataract blindness with the use of ECCE and posterior chamber lens implantation, unless inappropriate.

I believe that there is a strong incentive for implant surgery in the neglected rural communities as it is a challenge — it is new, unique and exciting and most importantly, it gives the patients excellent vision. In contrast, ICCE is an obsolete procedure — colourless and out of date and of little interest to most eye surgeons — even if successful patients have minimal vision from aphakia.

Eye surgeons, like other professionals, will respond more quickly to a voluntary organisation if such an organisation were run by eye surgeons, but not when it is a voluntary organisation of lay people where the eye surgeons, instead of being held as "experts" and essential, are regarded as mere "technicians". I believe that good response from eye surgeons will be most effectively generated by the creation of an international organisation of surgeons.

As the increasing importance of eye surgeons is now clear, we need to create incentives to attract them.

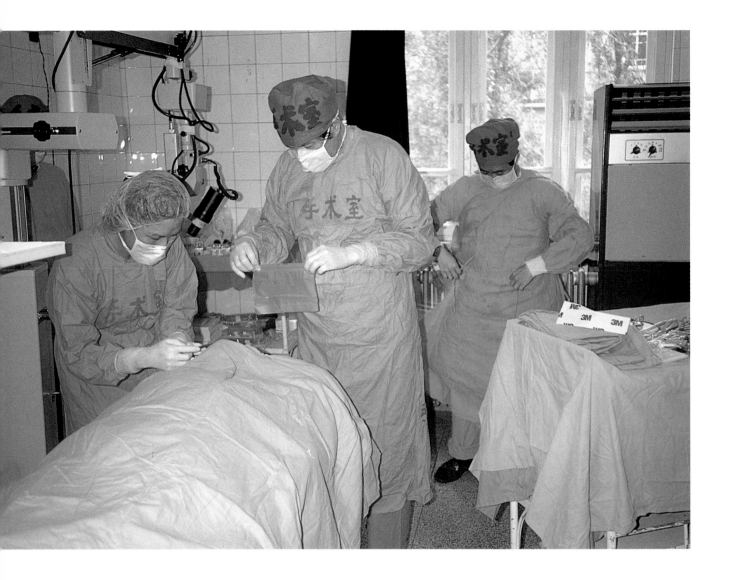

Dr Ang Beng Chong and Sister Peck Chye Fong were two pioneers with Professor Arthur Lim in Tianjin ten years ago, at a time when the world was generally against ECCE and PCI in developing countries. For the past twenty years, numerous courses on microsurgical techniques and implant surgery were organised by them.

Suitable Eye Surgeons

It is essential for eye surgeons to realise that the approach to cataract surgery in mass cataract blindness is different from that in the hospital environment. Mass cataract blindness, occurring in the poorer, neglected and rural communities of the developing countries, gives rise to a number of problems. These include problems of communication and transportation, lack of operating theatre facilities and operating microscopes, unreliable electricity supplies, lack of auxiliary staff, inadequate funding, the question of cost effectiveness, mass ignorance, danger of infection, lack of postoperative follow-up and facilities, etc. Eye surgeons have to perform surgery outside their usual hospital environment and this is a challenge. It requires adaptation to unusual and new situations.

Doctors are considered leaders and are looked up to by supporters and volunteers and by patients and their relatives. They must set a good example by their commitment and their understanding of the problems of the poor rural communities. They must also be sensitive to their cultures, traditions and religions. They are ambassadors. Unfortunately, some doctors are unsuitable as they are unable to adapt and should not be selected.

Organisation of World Eye Surgeons — WORLDCATS*

WORLDCATS (World Cataract Surgeons) has been proposed as an international movement of eye surgeons dedicated to the control of mass cataract blindness in developing countries, and especially in Asia, where millions are blind from this condition. As half of the cataract blindness is in Asia, this movement should perhaps be an Asian initiative.

It is a unique opportunity for eye surgeons to contribute their skills to help their fellowmen.

WORLDCATS has set up an initial target of 1,000,000 cataract surgeries, with implants unless inappropriate, over 10 years, through the organisation of 2,000 volunteer eye surgeons. WORLDCATS will also promote training and skills transfer in cataract surgical expertise to the developing countries. It will promote quality assurance in cataract surgery worldwide.

Funds and Support

Eye surgeons will contribute their time and skills for free. The funds

WORLDCATS (World Cataract Surgeons) is a unique opportunity for eye surgeons to contribute their skills to help their fellowmen.

*The name WORLDCATS has been changed to WORLDEYES to denote World Eye Surgeons Society.

for organisation, equipment and infrastructure will come from international voluntary organisations and foundations committed to the cause of alleviating mass cataract blindness.

Other Organisations

Cataract is a massive global problem which can only be solved by the combined efforts of organisations and eye surgeons.

To date, numerous organisations, for example, WHO, Lions International, Rotary Club, International Agency for the Prevention of Blindness, International Eye Foundation, Helen Keller International and many others have mainly tackled the non-surgical causes of blindness related to improving primary healthcare and have been using intracapsular extraction without implants in eye camps. WORLDCATS will complement the good work of these organisations.

Are there problems? Yes, of course, all major changes will encounter difficulties. But, I am confident of success.

Why WORLDCATS?

Why WORLDCATS, when there are so many international voluntary organisations already in existence? Why have another international organisation? In what ways can it perform better than the other established organisations?

The main and most cogent reason is the large-scale participation of eye surgeons whose services can be tapped for the benefit of their fellowmen. For years, the international voluntary organisations have not been too successful in recruiting sufficient eye surgeons. I believe that an international organisation of eye surgeons will generate stronger response from eye surgeons. An Asian initiative may be an additional stimulus for Asian ophthalmologists to respond.

Implant Training Centres

A major problem with visiting eye surgeons is its temporary nature. In the long term, the solution must be to teach the local surgeons to perform implant surgery well.

Adequate training will involve the teaching of basic microsurgical techniques besides techniques of ECCE and then the finer points of inserting a posterior chamber lens implant. From my experience, it will take half a decade to ensure that a group of surgeons, previously inexperienced in this technique, are trained adequately. As with other surgical skills transfer, the eye surgeons will learn at different speeds. They will need repeated exposure and interaction. Because of this, an important task of the visiting eye surgeons is to ensure sustained transfer of surgical skills and technology to the eye surgeons of the recipient country.

To train local implant surgeons well, the establishment of implant training centres, like the Tianjin International Intraocular Implant Training Centre in the People's Republic of China, with visiting eye surgeons actively conducting training and transferring skills and technology, is essential.

It is hoped that this Centre, in the next 6 years, together with other

> Adequate training will involve the teaching of basic microsurgical techniques.

> An important task of the visiting eye surgeons is to ensure sustained transfer of surgical skills and technology to the eye surgeons of the recipient country.

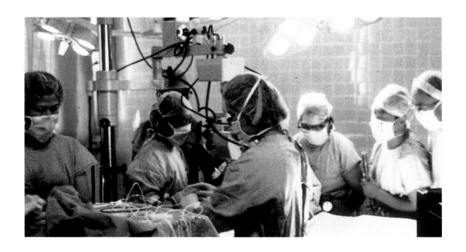

The courses emphasize teaching ECCE and PCI. This picture shows those in the operating theatre communicating via a two-way television system with participants in the lecture room.

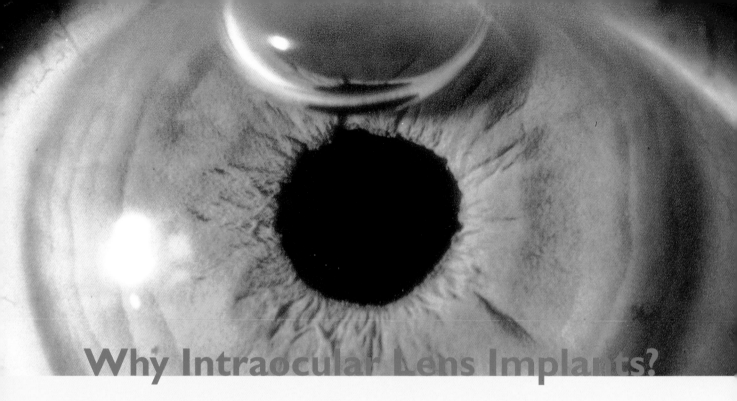

Why Intraocular Lens Implants?

I believe that implant surgery, unless inappropriate, should be the method used for the following reasons:

1. The visual results are superior.

2. Greater patients' satisfaction will encourage more patients to have surgery.

3. Surgeons' satisfaction leading to more contributions by eye surgeons worldwide.

4. Why deny our poorer fellowmen the benefit of implant surgery when it is achievable at low cost? Why use a method which is 30 years old?

5. Lens implantation in the rural areas is new. It is therefore an exciting challenge. ICCE has been used for decades without great success. It is like flogging a dying horse. The challenge of lens implantation will create interest as it is a new answer to an old problem.

6. Technical transfer and quality assurance is part of development.

7. It is achievable and the Tianjin International Intraocular Implant Training Centre is an example.

8. The unique opportunity of being part of a global movement aimed at restoring normal vision to millions of our less fortunate fellowmen.

centres in the People's Republic of China, will be able to perform or supervise 1,000,000 implants as demand spreads. The Tianjin International Intraocular Implant Training Centre may be a global model for all countries.

Conclusion

An organisation like World Cataract Surgeons is not just another international organisation. It not only confronts the problem of mass cataract blindness, it is a humanitarian organisation as well. It is about being humane, expressing our willingness to help the less fortunate. It is about international cooperation. It is a unique opportunity for eye surgeons to utilise their skills for the benefit of their less fortunate fellowmen. It is a challenge eye surgeons of the world should accept. In our troubled world, it can serve as a strong vehicle for international understanding and international peace.

There are few opportunities in the lifetime of professionals for them to — without disruption to their practice in any great way — utilise the skills they have been trained in to restore sight to millions of their less fortunate fellowmen.

It is a unique opportunity for all eye surgeons — worldwide. ✳

The Tianjin International Intraocular Implant Training Centre may be a global model for all countries.

An organisation like World Cataract Surgeons is not another international organisation... it is about being humane, expressing our willingness to help the less fortunate.... In our troubled world, it can serve as a strong vehicle for international understanding and international peace.... It is a unique opportunity for all eye surgeons — worldwide.

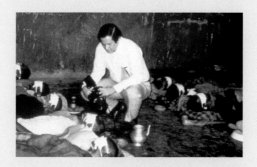

Quality Cataract Surgery in Rural Asia in the 21st Century

"Cataract blindness is spreading like wildfire to the rural poor in Asia: cost-effective ECCE and PCI can dramatically reverse the crisis of mass blindness."

Chapter 5

Quality Cataract Surgery in Rural Asia in the 21st Century

Professor Arthur Lim's keynote address at the 100th Anniversary of the Japanese Ophthalmological Society.

Introduction

The excitement of the "Information Age" has spread to virtually all major cities; and eye surgeons all over the world embrace its wide-reaching impact on every facet of everyday life. As a consequence, our professional practices will be radically different in the 21st century.

The spread of information and affluence to the cities has created fascinating contrasts within a nation. In India, the cities enjoy the benefits of modern housing, education and health services, similar to that in the developed nations, while the majority of India's population

Adapted from the Keynote Address delivered by the author at the 100th Anniversary Celebration of the Japanese Ophthalmological Society on 18 May 1996.

remain poor, living in the rural areas as farmers struggling against the forces of nature with poor housing and little education.

In the same way, the coastal region of the People's Republic of China enjoys standards of living approaching those of developed nations. Yet there are still hundreds of millions of Chinese peasants whose quality or way of life has remained unchanged. In Brazil, half-way round the globe, the situation is much the same.

While wealth and information have embraced all major cities of the world, they have failed to reach the world's rural population. Fortunately, in the past few years, conditions in rural Asia have been improving. In 1993, a World Bank study published under the title, "The East Asian Miracle", concluded that agriculture, while declining in relative importance, experienced rapid growth and improvement in productivity.

Political and Economic Changes

The affluence and spectacular economic development of countries bordering the Pacific Basin, combined with their ageing populations, will continue to increase the demand for quantity and quality of service from their ophthalmic surgeons well into the 21st century.

Political and economic changes have transformed much of Asia after the second world war. Before World War II, most of Asia was ruled by western powers who established empires that spread across the vast subcontinent of India to Burma and South-East Asia. The West dominated millions of Asians. The second world war had a dramatic impact on this state of affairs. The once invincible western imperial powers bowed to the whirlwind onslaught of Japanese military might that swept across Asia.

The conclusion of the second world war brought with it a strong wave of nationalism in Asia that resulted from the loss of confidence in the colonial powers. These events also had a dramatic impact on the practice of ophthalmology in Asia.

Under colonial rule, a local ophthalmologist, however brilliant and qualified, started and ended his career as an assistant medical officer. Under such conditions, local ophthalmologists simply stagnated given the lack of opportunities available to them. With independence and the departure of the colonial ophthalmologists, sweeping changes took place. From the 1950s onwards, thousands of ophthalmologists were trained. Thus the first important change in Asia was the emergence of vast numbers of Asian ophthalmologists.

The second major change was the economic progress in Asia. Most of Asia had, for centuries, remained poor. As colonies, their resources were exploited. It was the accepted way of life. In the past two decades, however, the area of greatest economic growth has swung from the countries in the Atlantic Basin to those bordering the Pacific Basin.

Tommy Koh (1995) reported that in the past few years, the world has experienced a change of historic importance. East Asia has risen in the world economy.

In 1960, East Asia accounted for only 4 per cent of world Gross National Product (GNP). In 1992, East Asia's share of world GNP went up from 4 per cent to 25 per cent. In Purchasing Power Parity (PPP) terms, East Asia's GNP was already larger than that of either the United States or the European Union, and by 2005, would be bigger than both combined. It was hard for many people in Europe and America to comprehend the reality that East Asia is, today, the new growth locomotive for the world economy.

The rise of East Asia in the world economy has either escaped the attention of many people in the West or has been greeted with disbelief because it has been so rapid and unexpected.

Thus the first important change in Asia was the emergence of vast numbers of Asian ophthalmologists.

Thus, the 20th century saw rapid political changes in Asia followed by great economic success.

The 20th century saw rapid political changes in Asia followed by great economic success.

East Asia's development has increased accompanied by the growth of per capita incomes (Table 1), the reduction of poverty and a fall in the infant mortality rate. The infant mortality rate of the United States (8.3) is higher than those of Japan (4.4), Singapore (5.0), Taiwan (5.7) and Hong Kong (6.4).

Table 1*

COUNTRY (1993)	PER CAPITA GNP (1996 forecasts in US dollars)	GDP PER HEAD (in US dollars)
Japan	$31,490	$40,500
Singapore	$19,850	$30,301
USA	-	$28,440
Hong Kong	$18,060	$27,040
United Kingdom	-	$20,490
Australia	$17,500	$20,200
New Zealand	$12,600	$17,230
Taiwan	$10,852	$14,470
South Korea	$7,660	$11,580
Malaysia	$3,140	$4,261
Thailand	$2,110	$3,110
China	$490	$520
India	$300	$335
Nepal	$190	-
Bangladesh	$220	-

*Source: Far East Economic Review Asia 1996 Yearbook and The Economist — The World in 1996

A third change influencing cataract blindness has been the increased lifespan of the Asian population.

A third change influencing cataract blindness has been the increased lifespan of the Asian population.

These changes will have a great impact on all aspects of life in Asia. In ophthalmology, the pattern of eye disease has changed. Major blinding conditions such as ocular infection and keratomalacia have decreased.

On the other hand, age-related blindness such as cataract, glaucoma and diabetic retinopathy are increasing. Cataract has surfaced as the major problem of increasing concern.

Have our approaches and techniques in the management of mass cataract blindness kept pace with this trend?

Quality Cataract Surgery in Asia

Cataract surgery has changed. Beginning with the operating microscope, multiple microsuturing, early mobilisation, ECCE and more recently, small incision extracapsular cataract extraction and phacoemulsification, these changes were initially regarded with curiosity and sometimes with skepticism. But it soon became clear that the new technologies centring around phacoemulsification and small incision cataract surgery produced excellent results. This created an enthusiasm not seen before. Thus, cataract surgery which was previously an uninteresting, colourless procedure, became an operation of immense interest.

It is against this backdrop that an unusual situation developed, which has schizophrenic overtones.

Many developing countries like India are burdened with millions of blind cataract patients in the rural communities. In these rural areas, even simple technology of eye camps is often unavailable, while eye surgeons of India's cities are moving rapidly towards phacoemulsification and small incision surgery.

Data on the number of cataract operations performed in Asia suggests that surgeons cannot even cope with the cases of new cataract blindness. As a result, the cataract backlog throughout Asia continues to grow, especially as the life expectancy in Asia continues to increase. Taylor (1995) indicated that only one out of six blind cataract victims has access to surgery. Cataract blindness in the world can double in ten

Cataract has surfaced as the major problem of increasing concern.

Cataract blindness in the world can double in ten years to 40 million because the world's population is ageing and we are not doing enough.

years to 40 million because the world's population is ageing and we are not doing enough.

Clearly, this trend creates a social and economic dilemma. On the one hand, developed nations and many major cities will enjoy all the advantages of modern cataract surgery. On the other hand, the poorer, neglected rural areas of the same developing nations face massive problems of delivering cataract surgery to the bulk of the population. It is in these parts of Asia where controversy rages over the choice of ECCE or ICCE and whether lens implantation is appropriate.

This is an unacceptable situation, and the world must react. As eye surgeons are now essential to the battle against mass blindness, we must lead.

Let us review the options available and formulate new plans for the effective delivery of eye-care in the 21st century.

Background

Many organisations have contributed to cataract blindness prevention programmes. One of the key players is the International Association for the Prevention of Blindness. Founded in 1929, it now has representatives from 28 countries and it evolved into the International Agency for the Prevention of Blindness (IAPB) on 1 January 1975.

Three years later, in 1978, IAPB held its first General Assembly in Oxford with Sir John Wilson as President. In the same year, WHO's prevention of blindness programme was established in Geneva. For the 18 years since, WHO and IAPB have held numerous meetings and have collaborated with numerous non-governmental organisations (NGOs) in developing programmes to prevent blindness throughout the world.

Important contributions were the microsurgical ophthalmic teaching workshops held regularly in Singapore and in Asia in the 1970s.

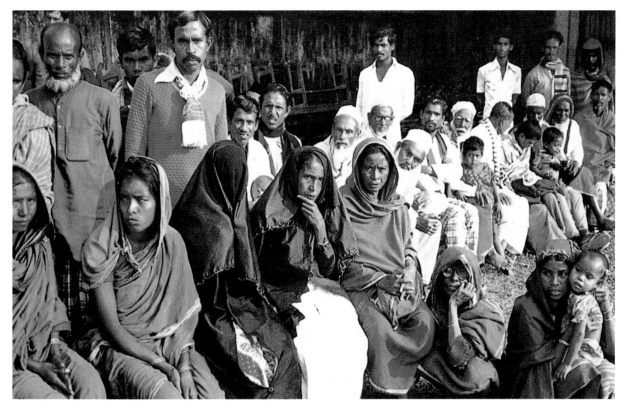

Crowd waiting.

These gave way to lens implant courses. Since 1986, implant courses
were held in the People's Republic of China. To consolidate and to provide continuity in such training, the International Intraocular Implant
Training Centre was built in Tianjin in 1989.

These activities in Asia culminated in 1990 with the ICO World Congress held in Singapore. Appropriately, its theme was the surgical prevention of cataract blindness. Akira Nakajima (1995), the President of
ICO, stated that the main theme "Surgical Conquest of Blindness" befit-
ted Singapore in the midst of developing countries.

At the end of the Congress, Rolf Blach (1990), Dean of the world
famous Institute of Ophthalmology, London, stated:

> *"... no doubt that the energy, the enthusiasm and the imagination of one*
> *man lifted the XXVI conference from yet another tired world jamboree to a*

mission to spread the word of the application of modern technological
ophthalmology to the underprivileged masses of the world..."

All this was six years ago. Action has yet to match the rhetoric to stem the rising tide of blindness from cataract.

Why are millions blind from cataract when vision can be easily improved? Why is ICCE still recommended? Is ICCE not obsolete, and should it not be replaced with ECCE and implants?

Cataract Blindness

It is a fact that after 20 years, with millions of dollars spent each month, the backlog of blindness from cataract has not been reduced. In fact, there has been a gradual increase as the number of cataract surgeries done per annum cannot cope with the number of new cases of cataract blindness.

This figure will continue to increase due to the lack of eye surgeons working in the rural areas of the developing nations. However, the number of surgeons is not the only issue — it is their training and the prevailing doctrines in eye-care delivery that have not met the challenges of modern times.

Let me illustrate the misery of cataract blindness by quoting a touching report by an Indian sociologist, Rajendra T Vyas (1990):

> *"While blindness from cataract is easily reversible, colossal numbers exist*
> *in the rural communities of the developing countries. The rural people wait*
> *helplessly for the day of deliverance from their miserable existence."*

Dr Vyas emphasized that millions are relegated to a life of utter dependency, destitution and degradation, living in misery and "condemned to a life of darkness".

Dr Vyas (1990) explained: "In many developing countries, there are inadequate or absolutely no old age pension or disability allowance scheme. Thus when that person becomes blind, he would be unemployed and has no means of supporting himself and his family. This results in starvation and early death and the family would become destitute."

He added that we have to ask ourselves whether "we are going to allow them to pass their days in darkness and destitution?"

The problem is sensitive and difficult but we must face facts. In the developing nations, millions of cataract victims remain blind and suffer from the horrible misery and socio-economic agony of blindness with no help and no hope.

If we do not act quickly, the numbers will continue to increase.

ICCE

The majority, two-thirds of patients operated on today in developing nations, are with ICCE — a 30-year-old method. Moreover, there are reports which indicate that the majority do not benefit from this surgery. ICCE done in eye camps at low cost without microscopes and sometimes with poor facilities has led to severe criticism because of poor visual results and high rates of complication.

Khalid J Awan (1987) stated that a careful study showed that only 50% derived any benefit. Another independent observer, Alfred Sommers (1990) confirmed this: "At least half of the people who have undergone allegedly successful surgery are blind, because they do not have aphakic glasses." Hugh Taylor (1995) also drew attention to the poor results of ICCE with only 25% obtaining improved vision results in some reports. In Saudi Arabia, the observation was that the complication rate of ICCE was 19%.

I have just returned from Nepal where there is a strong shift from ICCE to ECCE. I understand that in most Latin American countries, ICCE is now fading.

The majority, two-thirds of patients operated on today in developing nations, are with ICCE — a 30-year-old method.

Why is ICCE, which has been obsolete in developed nations for many years because of poor visual results, still recommended for the developing nations of Asia?

Politicians and governments should stop supporting an operation that is 30 years old. There must be incentives and rewards for eye surgeons, and we must change quickly from ICCE to ECCE.

Benjamin Boyd (1996) said: "If you refer to the World Atlas of Ophthalmic Surgery under HIGHLIGHTS, you might observe that not a single word about the intracapsular cataract surgery is mentioned."

Why is ICCE, which has been obsolete in developed nations for many years because of poor visual results, still recommended for the developing nations of Asia?

The reasons given to continue ICCE are: lower cost and it is faster to perform. In addition, there is the concern about an expanding backlog.

On the question of backlog, of course the backlog will increase if eye surgeons are not interested. They are not attracted to do ICCE. Why should they? It is an old method and it gives poor visual results. Furthermore, young eye surgeons today are not trained in ICCE . They are trained in ECCE with posterior chamber implant. This is a shame, because by sticking to ICCE, a greater backlog is created. Politicians and governments should stop supporting an operation that is 30 years old. There must be incentives and rewards for eye surgeons, and we must change quickly from ICCE to ECCE.

We must be frank and open. We must study the situation carefully, especially when we have failed to control blindness despite spending millions of dollars each month for many years. The problem is sensitive and difficult but we must face facts.

ECCE

It is well-known that the major cities and the wealthier communities within the developing countries will enjoy the benefits of technology, as they enjoy the benefits of better housing, education, communication and nutrition. It follows that patients who can afford to pay will demand quality cataract surgery. This has already happened in most developing nations in Asia because of growing affluence.

In the last few years, ECCE and PCI have spread extensively to almost all the cities of the developing nations. The demand for implantation has spread to the rural communities. It may take a few years. Communication and knowledge are powerful weapons. The rural population of the many developing countries will soon demand the best — ophthalmologists and politicians will have to meet the demand.

If we sit back and think, it will become clear that there is no physical handicap other than cataract blindness where normal function can be restored easily at low cost to millions. The excellent results of cataract surgery, compared with the results of help to the paraplegics, deaf and dumb, and the cancer and kidney patients, are unrivalled. It is clear that ECCE with implants is the most satisfying surgical treatment in the world.

In addition, ECCE and PCI will bring gradual advances in eye surgery to the developing nations. ECCE requires microsurgical techniques and with it, quality surgery will develop not only in cataract surgery, but also in glaucoma, in corneal surgery and in surgery of ocular injuries.

It has also been argued for some years that implant surgery encourages early cataract surgery, at a time when cataract patients are still working and are able to pay a small fee. This will attract more surgery and prevent blindness.

Dr Venkataswamy (1991) stated: "If we had given normal vision to them before they lost their jobs, their continued productivity and economic benefits would be a great asset for the nation."

Dr R.P. Pokhrel (1993) wrote that: " IOL enables cataract patients to return to their economic livelihood; more patients are able to contribute towards surgery and other programme costs."

Eye Surgeons

Many leaders have repeatedly stated that although the problem of

> Communication and knowledge are powerful weapons. The rural population of the many developing countries will soon demand the best

> "If we had given normal vision to them before they lost their jobs, their continued productivity and economic benefits would be a great asset for the nation."

cataract is difficult and well known, organisations have failed to control cataract blindness and support is inadequate. There are many reasons. One is the lack of response of eye surgeons. Let us study why the response of eye surgeons has not been good. Prevention of blindness has, for decades, been the role of nutritionists and public health workers. The surgeon's role was nominal. Furthermore, there was little incentive to attract eye surgeons. Why should an eye surgeon leave the comfort of his city practice to work in the rural areas where there is no incentive and no recognition? This must be changed.

As the importance of eye surgeons is now clear, recognition, honours and rewards are powerful incentives — we must create incentives to attract them. ECCE and PCI for mass cataract blindness is a strong incentive. It is new, unique and exciting and most importantly, it gives the patients normal vision. In contrast, ICCE is an obsolete procedure — out of date and of little interest to eye surgeons — even if successful patients have poor vision from aphakia.

Asia is growing wealthier. This growth will be more rapid as we approach the 21st century. I believe that the need for implant surgery in the developing countries in Asia is so compelling, it would be wrong to delay action. It would be wrong not to move forward.

Are there problems? Yes, all major and important changes will encounter difficulties and sometimes intense resistance.

How serious is resistance to change? We can recall in history the numerous frightening opposition to change and progress in medicine. It is unfortunate that some leaders directing cataract blindness continue to choose the comfort of cosy stagnation and oppose the progress of introducing low-cost ECCE and PCI in Asia.

Resistance to change is well known and has been the concern of celebrated American thinkers like Henry Kissinger (1985) and Milton

As the importance of eye surgeons is now clear, recognition, honours and rewards are powerful incentives — we must create incentives to attract them.

How serious is resistance to change? We can recall in history the numerous frightening opposition to change and progress in medicine.

Friedman (1980). I believe that a worrying danger to success is the smugness and arrogance of a few leaders who have closed their minds to new ideas and alternatives.

Eye surgeons from cities have to realise that the approach to cataract surgery in mass cataract blindness is different. Phacoemulsification is usually inappropriate mainly because of cost. There are sensitive issues relating to the infrastructure, culture, traditions and religion of the community. Unfortunately, some doctors are unable to adapt and should not be selected.

Another major problem is that visiting eye surgeons provide only short-term help. In the long-term, the solution must be to teach the local surgeons to perform implant surgery well. Adequate training will involve the teaching of basic microsurgical techniques besides techniques of ECCE. For surgeons with little previous experience, it can take many months. There is also the need for repeated exposure.

Tianjin

The establishment of implant training centres, like the Tianjin International Intraocular Implant Training Centre in the People's Republic of China, is effective for the training of local implant surgeons. As the problem is massive, it is important to establish more centres where national leaders, working together with foreign eye surgeons, can improve standards and teach their fellow ophthalmologists how to perform quality eye surgery at low cost.

In 1989, the Tianjin International Intraocular Implant Training Centre was formed and by 1996, it was clear that the concept was correct. This teaching centre has taught 1,500 ophthalmologists and has trained over 100 ophthalmologists for more than three months. In addition, it has established affiliated hospitals which work with the centre.

Altogether, the surgeons of the centre have now done 20,000 cataracts with ECCE and PCI, 8,000 in the centre and 12,000 outside the centre in the affiliated hospitals and regional hospitals. They plan to perform 100,000 operations by the year 2000, but hope for 250,000.

There is a well known saying that "If you operate on one man, you restore vision to one man, but if you teach your colleagues how to perform low-cost quality cataract surgery, they will solve the problem of cataract blindness in the world." This is the basis of our approach in Tianjin. I believe that if more such centres are established, there is hope that we can reduce and control the terrible problem of mass blindness affecting millions in Asia.

Modern communication will inform the world of the success of ECCE and implantation in the Tianjin Centre. It should be studied as a model for the developing nations as I am absolutely confident that it is the way we should go.

Future

Many requests have been made for this issue to be addressed. Hugh Taylor and Alfred Sommer (1990) made this request: "There is a need to address the issue of large-scale cataract surgery and to make a simple and safe ECCE and IOL surgery available in the areas where it is wanted. There are still a number of issues that need to be addressed and the time to address them is now." Alfred Sommer (1994) further stated that "there remains vast room for improvement."

International leaders frequently talk about human rights. Can it not be said that the restoration of normal vision to the blind of the world can be considered as the most important human right? Can it not be said that millions of cataract victims are denied the basic human right of normal vision? Are leaders of ophthalmic organisations guilty of failure

> "If you operate on one man, you restore vision to one man, but if you teach your colleagues how to perform low-cost quality cataract surgery, they will solve the problem of cataract blindness in the world." This is the basis of our approach in Tianjin.

> Can it not be said that millions of cataract victims are denied the basic human right of normal vision? Are leaders of ophthalmic organisations guilty of failure to take adequate action?

to take adequate action? Are we as eye surgeons guilty of omission, of failing to help and react strongly and effectively? Tianjin has succeeded. It will be disappointing if the rest of the world fails to move forward.

This move is about humanity — the willingness to help the less fortunate. It is about international co-operation. It is a challenge all eye surgeons should accept. This is important in our troubled world. It can also become a strong vehicle for international understanding and international peace.

Conclusion

When the human misery of millions of blind cataract victims continues to increase in the poor areas of our world, at a time when normal vision can be restored at low cost to all, we must press for action, for change. Let all eye surgeons of the world seize the moment. ✳

When the human misery of millions of blind cataract victims continues to increase in the poor areas of our world, at a time when normal vision can be restored at low cost to all, we must press for action, for change.

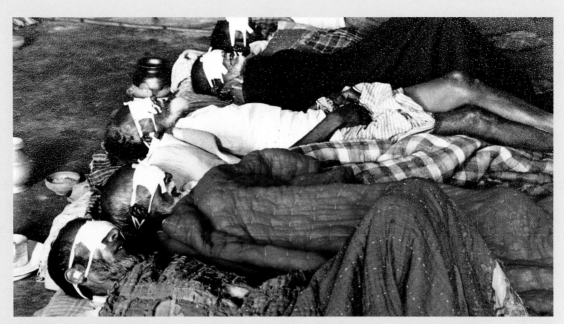

Post-operation

In developing countries, there are either inadequate, or absolutely no old-age pension schemes or disability allowance schemes. Thus, when a person becomes blind, he becomes unemployable and has no means of supporting himself and his family. This often results in gradual starvation and early death. The family then becomes destitute.

While blindness from cataract is easily reversible through surgery, the colossal numbers of cataract blind that exist in the neglected rural communities of the developing countries make it the world's major curable cause of blindness. While large cities and towns have facilities, the vast majority of people living in rural areas wait helplessly for the day of deliverance from their miserable existence. We have to ask ourselves whether we are going to allow them to pass their days in darkness and destitution? ‡

Rajendra T Vyas, 1990

Chapter 6

AMERICAN JOURNAL OF OPHTHALMOLOGY®

OCTOBER 1996
VOLUME 122

ORIGINAL ARTICLES

EDWARD JACKSON IN 1896: A MAN AND HIS SPECIALTY AT A CROSSROADS
LIII EDWARD JACKSON MEMORIAL LECTURE: PART I
Albert

THE VISUAL FUNCTION OF PROFESSIONAL BASEBALL PLAYERS
Laby, Rosenbaum, Kirschen, Davidson, Rosenbaum, Strasser, Mellman

VARIATIONS IN THE CLINICAL COURSE OF SUBMACULAR HEMORRHAGE
Berrocal, Lewis, Flynn

VISUAL FIELD LOSS IN HIV-POSITIVE PATIENTS WITHOUT INFECTIOUS RETINOPATHY
Plummer, Sample, Arevalo, Grant, Quiceno, Dua, Freeman

EDITORIALS

THE AJO: CONTENT AND CONVERSATION ON THE INTERNET AT http://www.ajo.com
Straatsma

EYE SURGEONS—SEIZE THE OPPORTUNITY
Lim

BRIEF REPORTS

RETINAL VEIN OCCLUSION AFTER TRABECULECTOMY WITH MITOMYCIN C
Dev, Herndon, Shields

CHOROIDAL NEOVASCULAR MEMBRANE
AFTER LASER-INDUCED CHORIORETINAL ANASTOMOSIS
Eccarius, Moran, Slingsby

MONTHLY SINCE 1884
Visit our Web Site and Authors Interactive™ at http://www.ajo.com/

AJO Centennial Meeting
Meet the Editors
AJO booth #4836
Oct. 26-Nov. 1

Eye Surgeons — Seize the Opportunity

American Journal of Ophthalmology,
October 1996

In conjunction with the American Academy of Ophthalmology Centennial Meeting,
28 October to 1 November 1996, Chicago, USA.

AMERICAN JOURNAL OF OPHTHALMOLOGY®

OCTOBER 1996
VOLUME 122

EDITORIAL

Eye Surgeons—Seize the Opportunity

ARTHUR S. M. LIM, M.B.B.S., F.R.C.S.

Chapter 6

EDITORIAL

AMERICAN JOURNAL OF OPHTHALMOLOGY, OCTOBER 1996

Eye Surgeons – Seize the Opportunity

"When human misery of millions of blind cataract victims continues to increase in the poor areas of our world, at a time when medical advances can restore normal vision to them at low cost, we will press for change, for action."[1]

Once in a century, a unique situation arises for eye surgeons around the world to contribute their skills to help mankind. Cataract extraction and intraocular lens implantation have been the major sight-saving triumphs of the 20th century, and now we find ourselves at another window of opportunity to improve the lives of millions of cataract victims in the 21st century.

As if to belittle the medical progress of the 20th century, the insidious might of disease continues, leaving millions blind from opaque lenses.[2] Mass blindness in the neglected rural communities of developing nations, has shifted from infection (onchocerciasis, trachoma, corneal

Reprinted from the American Journal of Ophthalmology, Vol. 122, Arthur S.M. Lim, Eye Surgeons — Seize the Opportunity, 571-573, 1996, with permission from Elsevier Science.

ulcers) and malnutrition (keratomalacia) to cataract. As lifespans have increased, age-related blindness from cataract now accounts for 50% of blindness in the world. Because only 20% of those blind from cataract have access to cataract surgery[1], mass blindness will double in number to 80 million persons within ten years.

In 1976, the world-renowned US futurologist, Herman Kahn, predicted that "200 years from now, we expect almost everywhere human beings will be numerous, rich and in control of the forces of nature."[3] Today, a mere 20 years after Kahn's assertion, human beings are already numerous, yet we are far from achieving universal prosperity, and are barely able to control earthly forces. However, one force which we do wield is our ability to restore vision to millions who suffer from cataract. The methods used are safe and effective, so why is mass cataract blindness still rampant?

The world is unfortunately complicated. The organization of nations has not successfully enabled the benefits of modern technology to be shared by people everywhere. Many leaders including Dr Bjorn Thylefors of the World Health Organization have reiterated their frustration that despite the acknowledgment of cataract blindness as a grave public health problem, an effective plan to resolve it remains elusive. The World Health Organization and the non-governmental organizations have helped but their efforts cannot keep pace with the number of new cataract victims. Thus, the backlog of millions will increase.

Dr Hugh Taylor reported in 1995 that five out of six of those blind from cataract die before they receive cataract surgery[4]. His estimate supports the contention that blindness in the world will double in 10 years. What can be done? How can we overcome this increasing chronic problem? In what way can eye surgeons help? What are the basic facts relating to this problem?

Since the 1960s, beginning with the introduction of the operating microscope, progress in techniques for cataract extraction has been extraordinary. Because of extracapsular cataract extraction, phacoemulsification, small incision surgery, intraocular lenses, and early mobilization, the patient with cataract-related blindness is almost always assured of normal vision within days of surgery. Such unparalleled successes (particularly compared with a previously colorless procedure of intracapsular cataract extraction) have captured the attention of eye surgeons throughout the world[1].

Driven by patient education and modern communication, this revolution in techniques has spread rapidly to the cities of the developing countries. Complete assimilation is but a matter of time as communication and comprehensive continuing medical education programs ensure that all surgeons will have the advantage of becoming adept at the new techniques. Accordingly, extracapsular cataract extraction with intraocular lens implant surgery is also reaching rural communities. Communication and knowledge are powerful weapons, and the rural populations of the many developing countries will soon demand the best services that can be provided.

If extracapsular cataract extraction with posterior chamber implant is the technique of choice, is the lack of trained eye surgeons in the rural communities then the limiting factor? Yes. Few eye surgeons are willing to sacrifice their urban practices to work in the rural areas or teach the rural surgeons. This problem appears insurmountable; incentives are lacking and sheer altruism is unconvincing as a persuasive argument. Governments, with international and national organizations, must recognize the contributions of eye surgeons who are willing to sacrifice time and money to help. Incentives and rewards must be introduced.

The answer lies in the training of eye surgeons who are willing to help for without these trained professionals, there will be no long term answer. The skills-transfer programs that are needed might take the form of highly focused special centers to provide the necessary training for rural eye doctors. Recently, such a novel experiment was successfully concluded, and its results are available for wider application.

Ten years ago, the concept of a training center was developed to teach extracapsular cataract extraction and posterior chamber implant was developed, and in 1989, the International Intraocular Implant Training Center (IIITC) was established in Tianjin in the People's Republic of China. Unlike other urban tertiary-care institutions, its main objective is not only to care for patients but also to graduate skilled ophthalmologists. With the cooperation of regional hospitals, it has been the training center for 1,500 ophthalmologists, and its programs have restored normal vision to 20,000 cataract patients in Tianjin and in the affiliated regional hospitals whose ophthalmologists were trained at this center. An ambitious plan has been launched by the IIITC; the aim is to perform 100,000 operations by the year 2000.

There are compelling reasons why the IIITC should receive our full support. We know from personal experience of no physical handicap other than cataract blindness in which normal function can be so fully restored, and at such low cost and with relatively little effort.

Compared with the treatment of paraplegia, hearing loss, cancer, and renal failure, extracapsular cataract extraction with posterior chamber implant has by far the highest value in terms of physician and patient satisfaction. Is this not one of the main reasons why we choose to be ophthalmologists in the first place? Furthermore, by requiring eye surgeons to learn microsurgical techniques, extracapsular cataract extraction introduces them to quality surgery, which will further benefit these practitioners in their glaucoma, corneal and ocular injury surgeries. Modern communications technologies will inform the world of the great success of the Tianjin Center. It will be a model for the establishment of other implant training centers in the developing nations.

This movement to alleviate cataract-related blindness should excite everyone, for it is about humanity: the willingness to help the less fortunate. It is about human organization. It is about international cooperation. It is a unique opportunity for eye surgeons and a challenge that eye surgeons around the world should accept. This is very important on our troubled globe; this movement can become a strong vehicle for fostering understanding and promoting peace worldwide.

International leaders frequently demand human rights. Can it not be said that the restoration of normal vision to an individual blind from cataract is a most important human right? Tianjin has succeeded; so have a few other centers, such as the Nepal Netra Joyti Sangh and the Aravind Eye Hospital in Madurai, India[5]. It will be disappointing if the rest of the world fails to sustain their success.

When information spreads, the need for eye surgeons will surface worldwide. The best way for anyone to help is to approach one of the many organizations involved, such as British Commonwealth Association for the Blind, Helen Keller International, the International Agency for the Prevention of Blindness, the International Eye Foundation, Lions International, Rotary International, World Cataract Surgeons Society and the World Health Organization. What greater value can eye surgeons have than to restore normal vision to the blind? All eye surgeons must embrace this statement: "A doctor's true wealth is the good he or she does for others in this world".

Let all eye surgeons of the world seize the moment, for it will not come our way again. ✳

Chapter 7

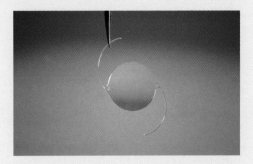

Changing World Opinion?

"In the 21st century, ECCE with PCI will become universally accepted as the procedure to restore vision to the victims of cataract blindness. This is because governments and leaders of the world can no longer close their eyes to the millions blind from cataract."

Chapter 7

Interview 1997:
Changing World Opinion?

The following interview is based on questions phrased by interviewers who supported the decision of several international organisations to use ICCE over ECCE for the rural blind of Asia. For one decade, they had been challenging the author's views on numerous occasions. The author explains his views that ECCE must replace ICCE as the surgical procedure for cataract blindness in rural Asia. To conclude, he holds up the Tianjin Centre in the People's Republic of China as a model of training and service excellence for the world to follow.

Interviewer

Why do you consider vision to be a human right?

Professor Lim

It is my opinion that of all the rights some leaders get excited about, the right for normal vision is the most important.

On 30 January 1996, the President of the International Agency for the Prevention of Blindness (IAPB), Dr Pararajasegaram stated:

The interviewer, Dr Ronald Yeoh, is Visiting Consultant at the Singapore National Eye Centre and Chairman of the Education Committee of the Asia-Pacific Academy of Ophthalmology

"I have reiterated our common contention that the right to sight is a fundamental human right and your endeavours in this direction are commendable."

Interviewer

Is it true that you resigned as Vice-President of the International Agency for the Prevention of Blindness?

Professor Lim

Yes. Ten years ago, when it was clear that there was disagreement with some key officers of the IAPB, I decided to resign from the important post of Vice-President to avoid internal dispute with colleagues who were also good friends of many years. They were strongly in favour of extending the use of ICCE for many more years, while I believed the solution lay in introducing ECCE and PCI worldwide as soon as possible.

It is clear that the visual outcome must always be foremost in the interest of our patients. It is wrong to think that because they are poor and uneducated, they need not have good vision.

One of the statements that disturbed me was, "These Asian patients are poor, illiterate and ignorant".

Interviewer

As an obviously ardent advocate for ECCE, is it possible that you have overlooked the benefits of ICCE? Why are you against ICCE?

Professor Lim

Every enlightened eye surgeon who has been actively performing cataract surgery would know that ICCE is not a satisfactory operation as the visual outcome is poor. Reports indicate that 50% remain blind after ICCE. Khalid J Awan (1987) stated that only 50% derived any benefit. Another observer, Alfred Sommer (1990) confirmed this: "At least half

I decided to resign from the important post of Vice-President to avoid internal disputes with colleagues...

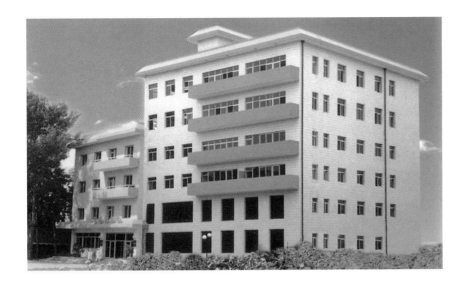

The International Intraocular Implant Training Centre Tianjin (IIITC).

of the people who have undergone allegedly successful surgery are blind, because they do not have aphakic glasses."

Just as important, ICCE has been considered obsolete because of poor outcome for years. We know that ECCE with PCI can restore normal vision and ICCE cannot.

Why is ICCE, which has poor results and is no longer used in developed nations, recommended for developing nations?

In addition, there has been tremendous economic growth in East and South-East Asia. In the cities of Asia, eye surgeons are moving to small incision cataract surgery, phacoemulsification and foldable implants. It is wrong not to move forwards into the 21st century.

It would be recorded in history as a serious error of judgement.

I wish to say that my comments are limited to Asia and I have left out other continents because I am not as familiar with their situations.

Interviewer

If ICCE is the only operation available, would you still recommend against its use?

We know the ECCE with PCI restore normal vision and ICCE cannot.

Supporting ICCE would be recorded in history as a serious error of judgement

Professor Lim

Let me put it this way. If the patient has no choice — as is the situation in some neglected rural communities, called the 'Fourth World' — then ICCE should be considered.

The situation where ICCE is the only procedure available is man-made — it can and should be changed.

Interviewer

You have explained the benefits of ECCE in your book, but have offered few solutions. Can you describe how ECCE can be implemented in the Third World?

Professor Lim

I have recommended that an alternative approach is to teach local eye surgeons to perform quality, low-cost ECCE with PCI.

The approach taken by WHO, IAPB and other international organisations have — after 20 years — not succeeded. We should look at alternatives. The estimate is that blindness from cataract may increase from 20 million to 40 million in the next 10 years. In addition, Taylor (1995) stated that only one out of six blind cataract victims receive surgery. The other five die without surgery.

Let us look at the People's Republic of China. The establishment of implant training centres, like the Tianjin International Intraocular Implant Training Centre, have been effective and rewarding.

The principle of my recommendation is based on teaching:

> *"Each time you perform a cataract surgery, you restore sight to one man.*
> *But if you teach quality cataract surgery to your fellow eye surgeons,*
> *you will restore sight to millions".*

In 1989, the Tianjin International Intraocular Implant Training Centre was formed and by 1997, it had taught 2000 ophthalmologists.

...an alternative approach is to teach local eye surgeons to perform quality, low-cost ECCE with PCI.

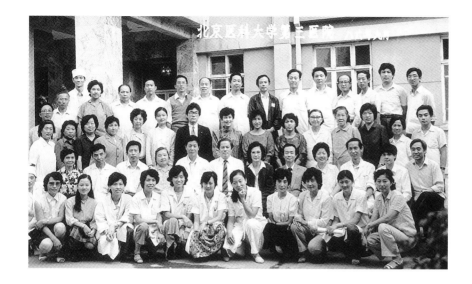

Ten years ago, regular teaching courses were started in the People's Republic of China. In 1986, Professor Arthur Lim ran an ECCE and PCI teaching course as the Honorary Professor of Ophthalmology, Beijing Medical University.

They hope, by working with other centres, to restore normal vision to 1,000,000 in five years.

Together with the other centres that are being built in Asia, 10,000 eye surgeons can be trained in the next five years. If each trained eye surgeon can do 400 cataract operations a year, 4 million cataracts can be performed each year.

I believe that this may solve the problem in Asia.

As the solution to mass cataract blindness is complex and difficult, I appeal for unity.

We must work together for success. What greater value can we as eye surgeons have, than to work together for the good of mankind?

The World Bank has permitted me to publish their exciting, outstanding and practical approach in India (letter of 11 June 1996):

"Key steps in India include:

(i) promoting a rapid change of technology towards the modern ECCE technique;

(ii) training ECCE with IOL of Medical College faculties in all seven project states, as well as over 1,500 government surgeons;

The World Bank has permitted me to publish their exciting, outstanding and practical approach in India (letter of 11 June 1996):

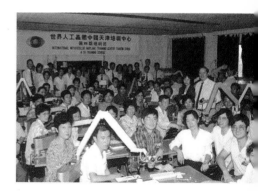

One of the many training courses organized by IIITC and attended by participants from all over China.

(iii) the involvement of private physicians already trained in ECCE / IOL, in partnership with NGOs and the government, to provide high-quality surgery to the poor, and

(iv) the construction and equipping of the facilities".

It is my hope that other donors will adopt the historic decision made by the World Bank.

Interviewer

Can you describe the role of training doctors to achieve the transition to ECCE and PCI?

Professor Lim

This is a very important question.

Trained national eye surgeons are essential for success.

I emphasize the importance of training centres and the incentive to have local eye surgeons properly trained. The International Intraocular Implant Training Centre in Tianjin is a very good example for the developing world to follow.

I have always argued that eye surgeons should be convinced that there is no greater contribution to mankind than the service of restoring normal vision to the millions blind from cataract.

The value of eye surgeons is to provide quality outcome at reasonable cost to their patients — especially to those who have little. Eye surgeons of the world — seize the moment — for it may not come your way again. (For more information, please refer to my Editorial in the American Journal of Ophthalmology 1996, Vol. 122, No. 4 in Chapter 6).

Interviewer

How would you answer your critics? Some have suggested that your recommendations have deprived blind people from minimum sight.

Professor Lim

Resistance to change is not uncommon. It is well known that many major medical advances in the past have been resisted, sometimes with great intensity. My critics should welcome the discomfort of honest disagreement as they are often a healthy sign of progress. A great error in life is the fear of facing errors and avoiding facts, especially when great misery to millions will continue. International organisations must acknowledge that they have failed after 20 years, and they should welcome an alternative approach. It would be wrong for us to continue congratulating each other at international meetings, year after year, while ignoring the fact that millions continue to suffer socio-economic misery.

I am surprised by their suggestion that I am depriving blind people of minimal sight. I ask: "Why are we restoring minimal sight to the blind of Asia when we can restore normal vision?"

I am disappointed with the international bureaucrats and their desire for cosy stagnation after 20 years of failure.

The Tianjin Centre trains many eye surgeons from the remote areas of China. I meet these eye surgeons whenever I participate in their courses and you should watch their enthusiasm when taught ECCE with PCI. They know this technique would enable them to give better vision to their patients. They are happy to learn an advanced and modern cataract procedure.

> My critics should welcome the discomfort of honest disagreement as they are often a healthy sign of progress. A great error in life is the fear of facing errors and avoiding facts

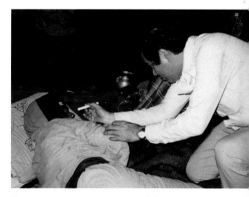

Examining a patient in an eye camp in India.

Interviewer

As you have stated, the transition from ECCE has already started, why is there a need to criticise ICCE?

Professor Lim

Time is the essence!

Each year we delay the transition to ECCE with PCI, is another year in which millions will have to suffer the misery and socio-economic agony of blindness.

I have kept silent for 10 years. I would be irresponsible if I continue to remain silent.

I would like the leaders of WHO to come out openly and discuss this issue concerning millions whose agony has been so poignantly described by leading Indian sociologist, Rajendra T Vyas :

> *"In developing countries, there are inadequate or absolutely no old-age pension or disability allowance schemes. Thus when that person becomes blind, he would be unemployed and have no means of supporting himself and his family. This often results in starvation and early death. The family then becomes destitute..."*

While blindness from cataract is easily reversible, colossal numbers exist in the rural communities of the developing countries. The rural people wait helplessly for the day of deliverance from their miserable existence. We have to ask ourselves whether we are going to allow them to pass their days in darkness and destitution?

Interviewer

Why are we delaying the transition?

Professor Lim

In countries where there are no infrastructure, what would you recommend as a solution to their mass cataract problem?

The 'Fourth World' communities in the neglected rural areas are in a sad situation. Cataract blindness is not their main problem. They have little education, poor housing, poor nutrition and poor basic health.

They only have one ophthalmologist to one million people. In these areas, ICCE may be the more appropriate approach.

I have kept silent for 10 years. I would be irresponsible if I continue to remain silent.

I expect this to be temporary in Asia as rapid economic progress is spreading to the neglected rural areas.

In 1993, a World Bank study published under the title, *The East Asian Miracle*, concluded that agriculture, while declining in relative importance, experienced rapid growth and improvement in productivity.

Communication, knowledge and public demand are powerful weapons. The truth will spread that ECCE can restore normal vision to the blind, but ICCE cannot.

Interviewer

If the use of ECCE with PCI increases operating time, won't the backlog of cases that already exists with ICCE worsen?

Professor Lim

On the question of backlog, it is my opinion that the backlog will increase if eye surgeons are not interested. You cannot attract them to do ICCE, why should they? It is an old method and it gives poor visual results. This is a shame, because by sticking to ICCE, more backlog will be created.

Politicians and supporters will stop supporting an operation that is 30 years old. People want to support procedures that give good results and if the results are not good, you will lose support.

Furthermore, young eye surgeons today are not trained in ICCE. They are all trained in ECCE with PCI. I wish to emphasise that we need the support of thousands of eye surgeons as we are dealing with millions of cataract victims. Where can you find thousands of eye surgeons to do ICCE?

I am quite certain that if WHO continues with ICCE, the backlog will worsen! In my opinion, there must be incentives and rewards and we must rapidly change from ICCE to ECCE.

It it an old method (ICCE) and it gives poor visual results. The is a shame, because by sticking to ICCE, more backlog will be created.

Interviewer

Is ICCE and anterior chamber implant an alternative? Would you accept this as a compromise to ECCE and IOL?

Professor Lim

If we are going to increase operating time, and increase cost and spend money on implants, why don't we be logical and move to ECCE with PCI? Why use a method which is known to give poorer results?

It has been known for many years that ICCE with anterior chamber implants results in more complications and poorer outcome. ICCE and anterior chamber implants are not used in cataract operations by reputable surgeons in developed nations and the cities of developing nations.

Furthermore, the basic principle of ICCE is wrong. Today's trend, set by the Americans, is towards small incision wound with phacoemulsification. All the advances of the 21st century will be based on the principle of ECCE.

With increasing affluence in Asia, phacoemulsification has already spread into the People's Republic of China and India. It is a negative move to introduce ICCE with implant.

Interviewer

Would the effects of posterior capsule opacification after ECCE and IOL negate the benefits?

Professor Lim

The problem of posterior capsule opacification is exaggerated. Most patients with posterior capsule opacification have a minor fall in vision. A minority develop more severe visual loss in three to five years. This is easily reversed with surgery or with the YAG laser. Furthermore, thousands of YAG lasers are already available in Asia.

There are many relatively minor problems like infection, cost, eyedrops, follow-up, outcome statistics, post-operative nursing care, transportation, etc. These are issues facing all nations. Although we need to address them, they must not cause us to deviate from the basic issue of restoring normal vision to blind cataract victims with ECCE and PCI.

Interviewer

In your opinion, what is the best portable microscope available, as there have been many complaints about the poor illumination of the microscopes used in the field.

Professor Lim

I do not think that microscopes pose a major problem. There are now many good low-cost microscopes with good illumination manufactured in developing nations. Excellent ECCE with PCI can be performed with these microscopes.

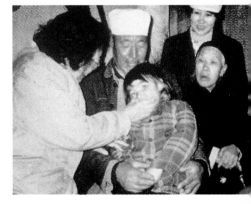

Prof JQ Yuan, Honorary Director of IIITC in the minority regions

Interviewer

It has been said that the centres that you build are located in the cities. As such, wouldn't it be difficult for the rural population to benefit?

Professor Lim

This is untrue. More than two-thirds of the patients receiving ECCE surgery in Tianjin, are from rural areas. More importantly, the objective of the training centres are to teach eye surgeons from the rural areas. They come from the district and village hospitals.

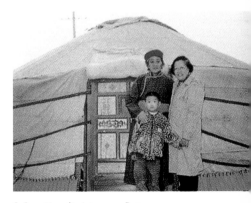

In Inner Mongolia Autonomous Region.

Interviewer

Why are you confident that the establishment of teaching hospitals, similar to the Tianjin Centre, will succeed?

Professor Lim

Success is based on good training and education. All the implant centres are designed for teaching. Success comes when everyone benefits. In performing ECCE and PCI, the patients benefit from normal vision; the surgeons are happy because of better results, and the hospitals, government, administrators and supporters are also happy. These are the essential factors for success.

In contrast, ICCE gives poor results. More than half the patients remain blind as they cannot see without glasses. And if they have glasses, they have difficulty getting about because of the visual dysfunction with thick cataract glasses. As a result, the patient is usually unhappy. The surgeons lose interest. In addition, eye surgeons today are not trained to perform ICCE.

Last year, I asked a young surgeon from South-East Asia who had just completed ophthalmic training: "How many ICCEs have you done?" I was surprised with the answer: "Professor, I have not seen one!"

Interviewer

Are there other blinding conditions that will become important in the future?

Professor Lim

Blindness from glaucoma — a condition of raised intraocular pressure — has become important. In addition, retinal diseases, especially diabetic retinopathy, is becoming a worrying cause of severe visual loss in many parts of Asia.

Interviewer

Ocular Surgery News, in their July 1997 issue, reported that your strong support for ECCE and your influence on foundations and the World Bank might have a negative effect for hospitals and surgeons who are doing ICCE. Will they lose the support of international foundations with the result that thousands of patients may not receive cataract surgery?

Professor Lim

It is my opinion that the victims of cataract will get greater support. They obtain better visual results. They are happy. The surgeons are happy. Governments, administrators and the public are happy.

Support comes when a move benefits everyone. The guidelines by the World Bank for the transition from ICCE to ECCE for India are outstanding and practical. I believe that NGOs, foundations and governments should follow the World Bank. This will generate even more support in the 21st century.

I appeal to international leaders to support this change as Asia is moving rapidly forwards and upwards into the 21st century with great excitement.

Interviewer

What do you predict will be the situation of mass cataract blindness in the 21st century? Can you, in one paragraph, describe the best approach to the prevention of blindness?

Professor Lim

The problem is complex and requires unity.

ECCE with PCI will become universally accepted. This is because governments and leaders of the world cannot close their eyes to the millions blind from cataract any more than they can close their eyes to the needs of housing, education, food, transportation and basic medical care. There is a saying: "it is easier to stop an invading army than to stop a good idea at the right time". ✳

Support comes when a move benefits everyone.

ECCE with PCI will become universally accepted

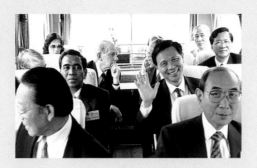

Ophthalmology in Asia Awakes!

"Asia, with more than half the world's blindness and half the world's population, is a continent of great contrasts. Burdened with poverty, ophthalmology remained primitive until recently because of economic progress and the determination of nations to provide all citizens with excellent eye-care. Asia has awoken to become the world's leading growth arena in medicine and ophthalmology."

Chapter 8

Ophthalmology in Asia Awakes!

"Ophthalmology in Asia, which has lain dormant
for centuries, will now awaken to a new dawn and rise up
to the challenges of the 21st century — Asia awakes!"

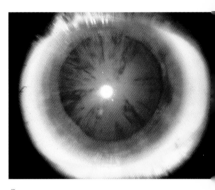

Cataract

For centuries, ophthalmology in Asia was mired in technological backwardness as its countries were plagued by poverty and dominated by imperial powers. In the last 50 years, Asian nations have become independent through the tireless efforts of great leaders. They have waded through seemingly insurmountable difficulties to carve a niche for Asia as a force to be reckoned with. With the effective erasure of colonial influence in this part of the world, Asian nations swiftly saw to the development of their economies. Today, Asia constitutes a formidable entity in the global financial market.

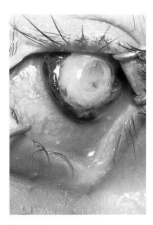

Keratomalacia

As a result of accelerated economic growth and an ageing population, the demand for quality ophthalmic care has surged. This, in turn, has brought about rapid developments in ophthalmology in Asia. However, prosperity has not extended to all the Asia-Pacific countries and advances in ophthalmology continue to lag behind in these countries.

Adapted from Daljit Singh Gold Medal & Oration, "Ophthalmology in Asia Awakes", delivered at the 10th ICIMRK Meeting, New Delhi, India, 1997.

Operating microscopes, intraocular implants and vitrectomy still reach less than five percent of Asia's massive population. Eye diseases caused by infection (trachoma and corneal ulcers) or malnutrition (keratomalacia) still prevail in poorer communities in rural Asia, leading to massive, preventable blindness. Furthermore, cataract continues to be the major cause of mass blindness because of longer lifespan and insufficient surgeons to remove the cataracts. Thus, more than half the world's blindness occurs in Asia.

Cataract continues to be the major cause of mass blindness... .

In order to avert the crisis of mass blindness in Asia, the more successful countries can assume crucial roles to improve ophthalmic care and research for the whole region. The close proximity and similar cultures and languages will enable quicker response to problems and provide a unique opportunity in the study of eye diseases which are influenced by race, climate and culture.

With mass blindness reaching almost crisis proportions in Asia, fuelled by the leaps that some Asian economies have made in training and technology, it would not be far-fetched to predict that by the end of the next decade, ophthalmology will emerge as the foremost medical discipline in Asia. The best doctors will be attracted to ophthalmology and the number of ophthalmologist will increase. Subspecialities will correspondingly develop. Witness the recent proliferation of eye centres of excellence throughout Asia. It can truly be said that ophthalmology has awoken in Asia.

Ophthalmology will emerge as the foremost medical discipline in Asia.

Asia in the 20th Century

Most of Asia has, for centuries, been held in the grip of poverty despite centuries of civilisation. Most nations in Asia were either under colonial rule or dominated by imperial powers.

The Second World War brought sweeping changes to this region.

The defeat of the British and Europeans by the invading Japanese forces in the Second World War was watched by Asians with great interest. When the impregnable British garrison in Singapore surrendered to the Japanese, it destroyed the belief in the invincibility of the European powers.

After the War in 1946, it was only natural that anti-colonial and nationalistic movements spread like wild fire throughout Asia. It was clear that it would only be a matter of time before Asia freed itself of imperialistic European domination.

How is all this related to ophthalmology?

In the early 20th century, in most of Asia, we had European doctors and local doctors. There were, however, major differences in their professional positions.

For instance, there were glaring differences in salary and advancement opportunities, but what was most upsetting was the vast difference in status. Under colonial service, a European doctor would begin as a medical officer. He would be assured of a rapid rise to the upper echelons of his profession. In contrast, no matter how brilliant and qualified he was, a local doctor would begin and end his medical career as an assistant medical officer. He stagnated in that position, and would never ever become a full medical officer.

With independence, the situation changed. Thousands of ophthalmologists were trained. And in the past 10 years, dramatic progress has occurred, mainly because of economic growth. First, in East Asia and then, South-East Asia and more recently, economic growth has spread throughout Asia.

> Under colonial service ... no matter how brilliant and qualified he was, a local doctor would begin and end his medical career as an assistant... With independence, the situation changed.

Asia Awakes

These changes all point to the dawn of ophthalmology in Asia.

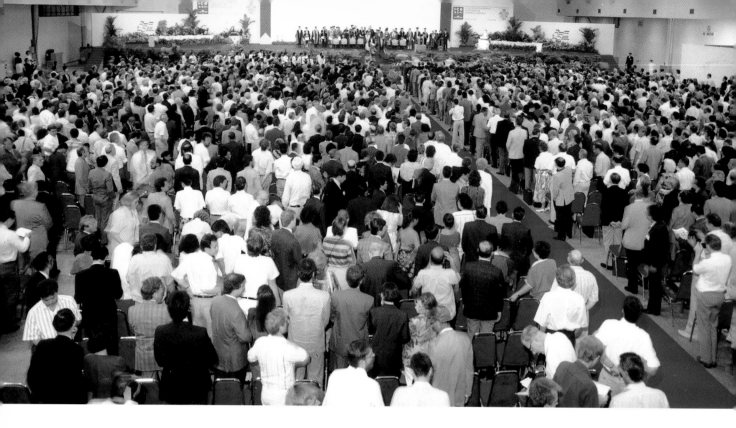

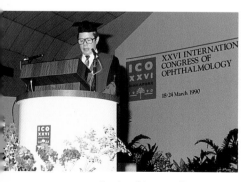

Some 8,000 participants from 81 countries at the 26th International Congress of Ophthalmology gathering at the official opening ceremony.

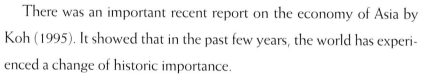

President of Congress addressing delegates.

There was an important recent report on the economy of Asia by Koh (1995). It showed that in the past few years, the world has experienced a change of historic importance.

East Asia has surged ahead in the world economy. In 1960, East Asia accounted for only 4 per cent of world Gross National Product (GNP). In 1992, East Asia's share of world GDP shot up from 4 per cent to 25 per cent. The purchasing power was, in 1993, already equal to that of North America's and Europe's.

With increasing purchasing power and rising demand for quality eyecare throughout Asia, especially in the cities, hundreds of manufacturers have converged on this region. These are just some of the indications that Asia, which has remained dormant for centuries, has awoken.

Are there any other indicators that ophthalmology has awoken? One of the most significant indications is the 1990 26th International Congress of Ophthalmology held in Singapore. Numerous participants declared that this was the most successful ophthalmic congress ever held in the world.

Let me quote some of the comments by the leading eye surgeons:

"....26th Congress has a profound meaning to all Asians and your effort made it possible that the Asian ophthalmologists can play a major role in the world ophthalmology community."
Saiichi Mishima
Emeritus Professor of Ophthalmology, Tokyo University, Japan

"It was really an immense success in every respect, and a delight for the participants. We all remember the general chaos at previous international congresses. Yours was a triumph."
P D Trevor Roper
Editor, "Eye" (Scientific Journal of the College of Ophthalmologists)
United Kingdom

"Of great importance for our Academy is the status you have given the region. I know this is a subject dear to your heart and how mightily you have succeeded."
Calvin Ring
President (1989-1991), Asia Pacific Academy of Ophthalmology
New Zealand

"You have established the standard for which all subsequent congresses must aim."
Stephen Ryan
President, Doheny Eye Institute
USA

"26th Congress has a profound meaning to all Asians.. ."

Saiichi Mishima

"Thank you for doing
the Asia Pacific
Region proud."

Ian Constable

"... no doubt that the
energy, the enthusiasm
and the imagination of
one man lifted the XXVI
conference..."

Rolf Blach

"... I decided to restart
these implantation
techniques after seeing
the excellent results
which Dr Lim showed."

Joaquin Barraquer

"Thank you for doing the Asia Pacific Region proud in Ophthalmology."

Ian Constable

Director, Lions Eye Institute

Perth, Australia

"...no doubt that the energy, the enthusiasm and the imagination of one man lifted the XXVI conference from yet another tired world jamboree to a mission to spread the word of the application of modern technological ophthalmology to the underprivileged masses ...."

Rolf Blach

Dean, Institute of Ophthalmology,

London, United Kingdom

"We are proud of you; you have certainly put Asian Ophthalmology on the World Map."

H J Merte

University of Munich, Germany

At the same Congress, Professor Joaquin Barraquer of the world famous Instituto Barraquer, Spain, speaking on lens implantation for cataract patients, stated:

> *"Until September 1989 we were observing, and I shall tell you that I decided to restart these implantation techniques after seeing the excellent results which Dr Lim showed."*

This is perhaps the first time that a highly respected world leader in ophthalmology has openly acknowledged the influence of the work of an Asian ophthalmologist. We should be proud — and humble.

From the 1980s, thousands of copies of ophthalmic textbooks by

Asian authors were sold in the developed nations. "The Colour Atlas of Ophthalmology" has also been translated into German, French, Finnish, Italian, Spanish and Portuguese. Who could have dreamt that the world would now be reading scientific and medical books by Asian authors? Indeed, the world is gradually changing its mindset.

Asia awakes: if we work together, Asian ophthalmologists will definitely set more trends in the 21st century. I am citing these examples to demonstrate the great influence of our work and achievements on the thinking of leading eye surgeons of other countries.

Furthermore, there is the emergence of leading eye centres throughout Asia — for example in Madras, Madurai, Hyderabad, New Delhi as well as Kuala Lumpur and Singapore.

Dr Keiki Mehta and his team have made dramatic moves by introducing phacoemulsification in the eye camps of India. Whether phacoemulsification should replace ECCE in rural Asia may remain controversial, but it illustrates an important point — Asian ophthalmic leaders are setting trends in ophthalmology.

In addition, many Asian leaders have argued that the use of ICCE by international ophthalmic organisations is wrong. Dr Keiki Mehta supports the use of phacoemulsification and implants. Many eye surgeons, including myself, have fought strongly for implants following ECCE. It is manifest that Asian ophthalmologists have taken the lead in the introduction of modern cataract surgery with better visual results for the prevention of mass cataract blindness in rural Asia.

Next, the seminal work of Asian researchers in relation to other eye diseases must also be highlighted.

Corneal research (Donald Tan, 1998) is rapidly progressing in Asia, especially in limbal allograft and amniotic membrane transplants — both of which are new forms of ocular surface transplants, pioneered largely

From the 1980s, thousands of copies of ophthalmic textbooks by Asian authors were sold in the developed nations.

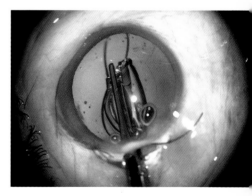

Posterior chamber implant.

by the corneal specialists of Asia; namely, Japan, Singapore, Australia, Taiwan, Thailand and Korea.

In glaucoma, clinical trials have shown that the use of Argon laser iridoplasty is an effective way to treat acute angle closure glaucoma, especially in situations where the response to medical therapy is poor. These findings have not only been published in international journals, but are also now a reference in the major textbooks on glaucoma.

In addition, Asian ophthalmologists (Steve Seah, 1998) are amongst the pioneers in the research on the modulation of glaucoma wound healing to improve the success of trabeculectomy. C W Chen from Taiwan was the first to use Mitomycin-C in trabeculectomy. A major clinical trial on the use of 5-Fluorouracil is currently being conducted at the Singapore National Eye Centre.

Over 15 years ago, lens implantation in patients with diabetic retinopathy was considered wrong. Western ophthalmologists (Drews & Steele) stated: "Sick eyes do not make good homes for implants." Asian ophthalmologists argued against this and asked: "If implants give cataract patients such good vision, why are diabetics denied this great advance?" Numerous related articles have also been published by Asian authors in international journals.

Today, 15 years later, it is quite clear that patients with diabetic retinopathy should not be denied lens implantation.

Teaching courses (Ronald Yeoh, 1999) by Asian eye surgeons are held throughout Asia extending to USA, Europe and Australia. There are many more examples — all indicating that ophthalmology has awoken in Asia.

Trends

Over the past decades, Asia has been obsequiously following the trends

> "If implants give cataract patients such good vision, why are diabetics denied this great advance?"

of Europe and USA. By the year 2000, the situation will change. Asia will be the trendsetter. It is therefore important for us to study the existing trends in the different nations of Asia.

Trends in Europe and USA

In the 20th century, North America prospered and established major eye institutes. In the last 3 decades, these centres have influenced subspecialisation, teaching as well as clinical and basic research throughout the world. North America has been setting the trend for every field of medicine, including ophthalmology.

General Trends in Asia

In the last decade, however, the world has seen the emergence of Asian influence in many aspects of contemporary life.

In the legal field, for example, the jury system was demolished in many Asian countries. Death sentencing for drug traffickers and mandatory caning was introduced. These swiftly became international controversies amidst allegations of human rights abuse. Yet many cities in Asia have become safer than New York, London or Sydney. A distinctively Asian set of human values have also emerged. The strengthening of family ties, respect for leaders, press restriction and censorship of films with undesirable sex and violence are just some examples of the move away from North-American and European influences.

A distinctively Asian set of human values have also emerged.

Ophthalmology in Asia

In medicine, Asia is constantly looking for ways to avoid high costs. We are concerned that the North-American system is heading for health costs higher than 13% GNP, compounded by legal suits and the almost limitless explosion of new, costly technology and procedures. We note that even the government of USA (the richest country in the world), has taken steps to control spiralling health costs.

It is therefore not surprising that in Asia, governments, hospitals and medical practitioners are looking into cost-effectiveness, questioning new, costly procedures and technology and finally, arguing that the latest may not be the best.

Thinking patterns will change. The 21st century will mark a turning point in the mindsets of Asian eye surgeons: they will analyse and follow the trends of Asian nations instead.

The 21st century will mark a turning point in the mindsets of Asian eye surgeons: they will analyse and follow the trends of Asian nations instead.

Admiration for Western Achievements

Let me emphasize that I have the greatest admiration for European and American achievements in innovations and technology. In fact, Asian doctors need to study the Mayo Clinic's philosophy of compassion towards patients, where every patient is made to feel that he is important and given the greatest consideration in the management of his condition. Other aspects of American professional etiquette worthy of emulation are the spirit of cooperation and unity as well as the recognition and promotion of excellence. Just as the Americans honour top achievers like the Mayo doctors, Harold Scheie and Edward Maumanee, we too should single out our most competent doctors for praise.

... there is a strong trend for commercial firms to support ophthalmic meetings throughout Asia. This will grow, once the financial setback in Asia is over.

Ophthalmic Congresses and Meetings

With the increased demand for quality eye-care and growing purchasing power in Asia, there is a strong trend for commercial firms to support ophthalmic meetings throughout Asia. This will grow, once the financial setback in Asia is over.

Realising this, the American Academy of Ophthalmology, by inviting more Asians to be members of the Academy, aims to attract more

Asians to attend their congresses. And as for the Association for Research in Vision and Ophthalmology (ARVO), 50% of the participants are Asians.

Why are these observations important?

Within 10 years, the participation of Asians in international meetings like the American Academy and the ARVO will decline as more meetings will be held in Asia. This is already happening as eye meetings throughout Asia have, in the past few years, continued to generate strong support.

One can credibly say that in the new millennium, Asia will be the cynosure of world developments.

At the same time, it is important that Asian ophthalmologists not only work in unity, they must also cooperate with their colleagues of Europe, America and Australia. We must recognize that numerous European, Australian and, in particular, American ophthalmologists have been very generous in training Asian ophthalmologists over the past decades. The only difference is that Asia has awoken, and we will work together as equal partners.

21st Century

With the advent of the 21st century, various aspects of the ophthalmic profession will be brought into sharp relief.

For instance, the challenge of providing cost-effective eye-care to the rural poor will have to be tackled. Next, other issues at stake are: what is the value of phacoemulsification in rural Asia? Is there a cheaper substitute for Healon? Can the cost of implants be lowered? Should surgeons spend hours trying to restore limited vision in eyes with badly damaged retinas?

Then, there are the questions on quality assurance. Should not a

... in the new millennium, Asia will be the cynosure of world developments.

one-eyed patient be operated on only by the best surgeons? How can surgical skills be measured? What will be the scenario of ophthalmology in Asia-Pacific in the year 2010?

By the year 2010, I believe that the following changes will take place:

- Ophthalmology will emerge as the foremost surgical discipline. This will come with escalating demand for quality treatment as sight becomes more important with education, the requirements of good vision for television and computers, and an ageing population.
- The best doctors will be drawn into ophthalmology.
- There will be a two-fold increase in the number of ophthalmologists in response to increasing demand.
- Subspecialisation will be firmly established. We will have retinal surgeons, pediatric ophthalmologists, oculoplastic surgeons and those specialising in glaucoma and so on.
- More major eye centres will develop, working in close co-operation and complementing one another, and all aiming for international excellence.
- The private sector will play an increasingly important role in major ophthalmic developments. By virtue of the rapid changes, it is more likely that private enterprises will lead in development. It is well known that governments and large organisations tend to move more slowly.

These changes will lead to a higher standard of eye-care, and with it, hopefully, a fall in the incidence of blindness.

In our enthusiasm to meet increasing demand, we must not forget to address the problem of cost. We need to choose carefully the numerous new equipment, for the latest may not necessarily be the best.

The future for ophthalmologists in Asia bodes well: they have the

By 2010... there will be escalating demand for quality treatment as sight becomes more important exciting opportunity, as never before in the history of medicine, to provide our people with world class eye-care.

Cataract Surgery in Rural Asia

Despite the burgeoning developments of recent years, the crisis of mass blindness still looms ahead for rural Asia. Fortunately, the economic growth of East Asia and other major cities is gradually spreading to these areas.

In 1993, a World Bank study published under the title, "The East Asian Miracle", concluded that in East Asia, agriculture, while declining in relative importance, has experienced rapid growth and improvement in productivity.

Eventually, rural Asia will awaken: light is spreading throughout rural Asia. A notable example is the Aravind Eye Hospital in Madurai, India. Under the capable leadership of Dr Venkataswamy, normal vision with ECCE and posterior chamber implants is being restored to thousands of patients each month.

Another exciting indication that light shines in India is the loan of over US$100 million by the World Bank to the Indian government. I expressed my delight in my correspondence and discussion with World Bank officials, including the President of the World Bank.

The World Bank, in a letter of 11 June 1996, indicated that if all goes well, India hopes to provide surgery to 11 million cataract victims. I also had a discussion with one of the most outstanding leaders of India, the Minister of Commerce, Mr Chidambaram.

Mr Chidambaram has been involved with cataract blindness work in India for many years, and was full of enthusiasm and determination about the progress in India. I was honoured to receive the Malik Gold Medal from him in 1992.

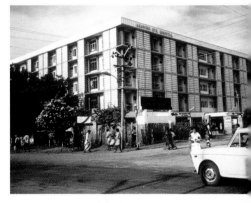

The Aravind Eye Hospital of India.

Eventually, rural Asia will awaken: light is spreading throughout rural Asia.

Asia-Pacific Journal of Ophthalmology Vol 12 No 2   April 2000

EWS

Since its inception in 1958, the Asia-Pacific Academy of Ophthalmology (APAO) has made tremendous progress in its mission against major blinding diseases in the Asia-Pacific region. Its success is due in no small part to the dedication and good faith of its members who have pooled together their experiences, ideas and expertise to spread the benefits of modern eye-care to their fellowmen.

When the first Asia-Pacific Congress was held in Manila 40 years ago, only 128 delegates from 12 countries were in attendance. 40 years later, the congress has returned to the same venue, but with a major difference: the 17th Congress in Manila, Philippines, March 7-12, 1999, saw a spectacular turnout of 1000-odd delegates coming from 18 member countries. They participated enthusiastically in the scientific programme - consisting of 14 symposia, 23 instructional courses, 17 special lectures, 238 papers, 52 scientific posters, and 20 video presentations – all of which leaned towards various concerns for eye-care in the next millennium.

Highlights of the congress included the Susruta lecture on "A global approach to cataract intervention" delivered by the incoming APAO president, Professor Mohammad Daud Khan, M.D., and the presentation of the Jose Rizal Medal as well as the Jose Rizal Gold Medal to Professor Sang-Wook Rhee, M.D., Korea, and Professor Joaquin Barraquer, M.D., Spain, respectively.

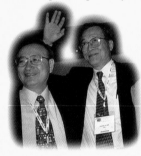

Prof Te-Tsaw Chen and Prof J H Liu, Executive Committee members of the 18th APAO Congress, Taipei 2001.

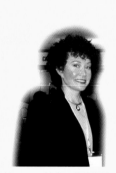

Dr Marguerite McDonald (USA).

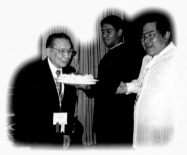

Sharing the joy with birthday boy, Dr Romeo Fajardo (17th APAO Congress President), is Dr Antonio Say (white shirt) of Philippines.

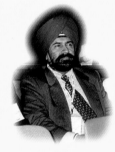

Dr Pall Singh, Malaysia (APAO council member)

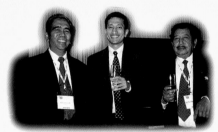

Three Cheers from the doctors - Prof Mardiono Marcetio (Indonesia), A/Prof Vivian Balakrishnan (Medical Director, Singapore National Eye Centre) and Dr Ram Prasad Pokhrel (Nepal).

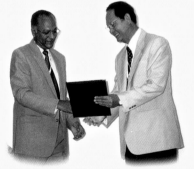

Prof S Selvarajah (Immediate Past-President of APAO) receiving the certificate for delivering the Holmes Memorial Lecture by Prof Prachak Prachakvej (President, APAO).

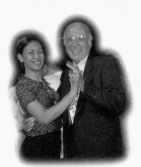

Prof Joaquin Barraquer (Director, Barraquer Institute, Spain) puts on his dancing shoes.

Asia-Pacific Journal of Ophthalmology Vol 12 No 2   April 2000

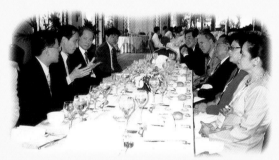

A business lunch at the Manila Hotel with officials from China. (Left, front to back – Mr Zhang Guozhong and Deputy Director of CDPF, Mr Liu Xiocheng, Vice Chairman of CDPF, Prof A Lim, Mr Lai Wei, Deputy Director of CDPF. Right – Dr Pearl Tamesis-Villalon, President, Philippine Academy of Ophthalmology, Mrs A Lim, Dr R Fajardo, Prof Daud Khan (In-coming President, APAO) and Mr Wu Minjiang, Director General of Ministry of Health, China.

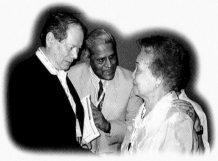

Prof A Lim, Secretary General, APAO with Mr Liu Xiocheng, Vice Chairman, China Disabled Persons' Federation (CDPF), Secretary General of "SightFirst China Action" Chinese Executive Committee.

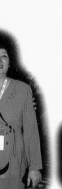

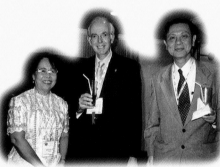

The gracious host, Dr Gloria D Lim (Adviser to the Organising Committee of the 17th APAO Congress) with Dr Frank Martin, Chairman, Division of Surgery, Royal Alexandra Hospital for Children, Australia and Prof Por T Hung, Chairman of the forthcoming 18th APAO Congress 2001, Taipei.

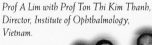

Prof A Lim with Prof Ton Thi Kim Thanh, Director, Institute of Ophthalmology, Vietnam.

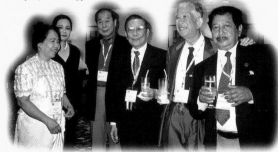

A private function hosted for council members. (From left: Dr Gloria Lim, Dr Pearl Tamesis-Villalon, Dr Lim Kuang Hui (Singapore), Dr R Fajardo, Prof Akira Nakajima (Past Secretary General, APAO) and Prof Ram P Pokhrel (Nepal).

Sharing sweet memories were Mrs De Ocampo (Philippines), Prof A Lim and Dr SS Badrinath (India).

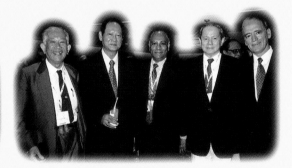

A handsome snapshot of Presidents and Secretary-generals of APAO (From left:- Prof A Nakajima, Prof P Prachakvej, Prof S Selverajah, Prof A Lim, Prof D M Khan.)

"The health specialists in the Bank's India Country Department... fully agree that ICCE (intracapsular cataract extraction) is an obsolete method for cataract surgery.... We applaud this historic move by the World Bank, working together with the Indian government."

In a letter of 11 June 1996, the World Bank made a most important statement:

"The health specialists in the Bank's India Country Department, who were responsible for appraising the Government of India's Cataract Blindness Control Project, fully agree that ICCE (intracapsular cataract extraction) is an obsolete method for cataract surgery.

In fact, the Cataract Blindness Control Project has, as one of its key objectives, the promotion of a transition from ICCE to the modern procedure of Extracapsular Cataract Extraction (ECCE) with intraocular lenses (IOL).

This transition, as you undoubtedly appreciate, requires some years to fully accomplish.

In addition to promoting the technological change to ECCE with IOL, the project will make it possible to carry out about 11 million surgeries which will restore sight to millions of poor blind people in India.

Without the support from the World Bank for the project, India would have continued to accumulate a growing backlog of cataract blind, at a significant economic and social cost to the country."

We applaud this historic move by the World Bank, working together with the Indian government.

Next, light is also spreading in the People's Republic of China. Ten years ago, the International Intraocular Implant Training Centre in Tianjin was built. It has achieved spectacular success. This centre has trained 2,000 eye surgeons to perform low-cost quality ECCE and PCI. With the International Intraocular Implant Training Centre as a model, five more centres have been built in China. Plans are being made to build 10 such centres in Asia.

There is a well known saying: "If you operate on one man, you restore vision to one man, but if you teach your colleagues how to perform low-cost quality cataract surgery, they will solve the problem of cataract blindness in the world".

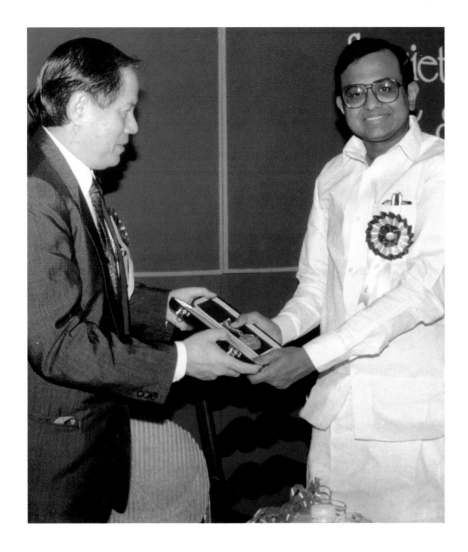

*Receiving the Malik Gold Medal from the
Minister of Commerce of India,
Mr Chidambaram in New Delhi,
13 March 1992.*

This is the basis of our approach in Tianjin. I believe that if more such centres are established, there is hope that we can reduce and control the terrible problem of mass blindness affecting millions in Asia.

The enthusiasm of China and the plans of India are exciting as they indicate that we may begin to solve the problem of cataract blindness in rural Asia by the year 2000. However, such projects provoke the following concerns: can we train enough surgeons? How do we keep the costs low? How do we ensure good visual outcome?

In spite of these thorny issues, the future looks promising. The fact

The fact that the World Bank has affirmed that ICCE is obsolete and that the Tianjin Centre teaches ECCE, ignoring ICCE, are essential steps to fulfilling our long-term vision.

that the World Bank has affirmed that ICCE is obsolete and that the Tianjin Centre teaches ECCE, ignoring ICCE, are essential steps to fulfilling our long-term vision.

Above all else, I appeal for unity - let us work together to attain our goals for quality world vision.

"When the human misery of millions of blind cataract victims continues to increase, at a time when normal vision can be restored at low cost, we must press for action, for change."

Renaissance (Rebirth)

It is clear that with affluence, efficient organisation and eminent leadership, ophthalmology will achieve resounding success across Asia. As we enter the next millennium, let us not forget the ground-breaking work of our ancestors. The genius of an Asian ophthalmologist comes to mind. Susruta, a native of ancient Bangladesh, was an ophthalmologist around 1000 BC.

He was not only the greatest exponent of treating cataract with couching, but he also described with surprising accuracy the anatomy, physiology and pathology of the eye. Each day, Susruta would fumigate his operating room with sulfur fumes and incense. Sulfur dioxide gas is a well known antiseptic and detergent, and incense fumes contain essential oils which also have antiseptic properties.

Before proceeding with an operation, he would take a bath and change his clothes, cut his nails as well as have his long hair tied in a knot on top of his head. Susruta knew that preoperative cleanliness would minimize postoperative complications.

In this, he was hundreds of years ahead of the British and European eye surgeons. He is a legend amongst numerous other Asian leaders in ophthalmology.

Outstanding Asian Ophthalmologists

National Hero of the Philippines
Jose Rizal

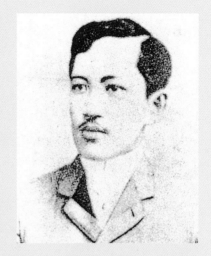

Jose Rizal

(1861 - 1896)

Jose Rizal was not only the national hero of the Philippines, but also an ophthalmologist by training and profession.

After completing his medical studies at the Central University of Madrid in Spain, he went on to receive training in ophthalmology under the famous leaders of the day — Louis de Wecker (Paris) and Otto Becker (Heidelberg).

Upon returning to his native country, the Philippines, he devoted himself to ophthalmic and political pursuits — he was driven by a consuming urge to plant the seeds of national ophthalmology in the Philippines as well as to emancipate his people.

Throughout his career, his ophthalmic practice was beset by difficulties and trying circumstances. Yet his clientele was huge and varied, coming from all parts of his native country and the world. Similarly, his political life and life as a revolutionary figure are legendary. At the age of 35, he was executed by the Spanish colonialists for his pro-patria activities.

Rizal's place in the history of Filipino ophthalmology is secure. He was the first well-known Filipino ophthalmologist, if not the first Filipino to take up postgraduate studies on eye diseases abroad. He was also the pioneer of ophthalmological practice in his native country. To commemorate his pioneering role in ophthalmology, "The Jose Rizal Award for Excellence in Ophthalmology" was proposed in 1964, and the first award was given out in 1968 to Dr Geminiano de Ocampo from Germany.

It may truly be said that Jose Rizal was the pioneer Filipino ophthalmologist, a beacon of light and an inspiration to the present and future generations of Filipino ophthalmic surgeons, physicians and medical students.

*Adapted from "Ophthalmology Awakens in Asia —
40 Years of Asia-Pacific Ophthalmology" (1999).*

Discoverer of the Trachoma Virus

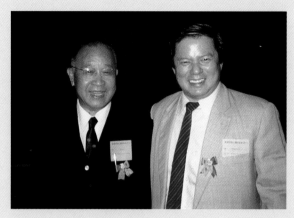

From left: Professor Zhang Xiao-lou with Doctor Arthur Lim

The late Professor Zhang Xiao-lou

(China) BS, MD (1914 - 1990)

The world will remember Zhang Xiao-lou as the ophthalmologist who, together with the virologist Professor Tang Fei-fan, were the first in 1954 to cultivate the virus of trachoma — an ancient disease still rampant in the Third World. Their success in the cultivation of trachoma bodies in chick embryo, after many futile efforts by other research workers worldwide, was a signal triumph in basic research by Chinese scientists — an epoch-making breakthrough that paved the way for meaningful research in this field.

In recognition of his discovery and his later work on trachoma, Professor Zhang received many international and national awards and appointments, among them the Award of Merit, National Symposium of Science and Technology in 1978 and a gold medal from the International Prevention of Trachoma Association in 1981.

Following his pioneering work on trachoma in 1954, he was appointed the deputy director and finally director of the Beijing Eye Research Centre (the first basic research facility to be established in China), an appointment he held until 1985. From 1950-1965, he was also associate professor and finally professor of ophthalmology at the Shuei He Medical College (his alma mater).

When Professor Zhang passed away in Beijing, PRC, in September 1990 at the age of 76, his death was mourned by the Beijing Tong Ren Hospital (where he was still at work as its deputy director), as a "great loss to our country's ophthalmology and a loss to the whole country's technical field". History will record his spectacular achievements, and the name of Zhang Xiao-lou, coupled with Tang Fei-fan, is secure in the literature for pioneering work on trachoma. It speaks much of their accomplishment that 40 years after their discovery, a vaccine for trachoma has yet to be found, in spite of intense research efforts worldwide.

Adapted from "Ophthalmology Awakens in Asia — 40 Years of Asia-Pacific Ophthalmology" (1999).

The Eye Surgeon of the 20th Century

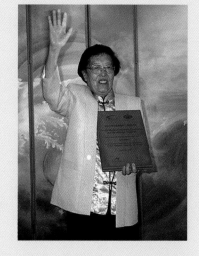

Professor Yuan Jia-Qin

(1919 -)

Professor Yuan Jia-Qin, clinical professor of ophthalmology in Tianjin Medical University, is the founder, ex-director and current Honorary Director of the International Intraocular Training Centre (IIITC) in Tianjin, China.

Since 1978, Professor Yuan has received numerous national medals and honours from international organisations for her vital contributions to the development of ophthalmology in China and the world. Her international awards were presented by the Asia-Pacific Academy of Ophthalmology (1987), XXVI International Congress of Ophthalmology (1990) and Singapore National Eye Centre (1993), amongst others.

Since the Tianjin Centre was successfully initiated and established by Professor Yuan a decade ago, implant surgery has developed widely and rapidly in China. With the use of ECCE and PCI, she has restored normal vision to 120,000 blind cataract patients in the People's Republic of China, and plans to restore normal vision to 1,000,000. Under her effective leadership, 2,250 ophthalmologists were trained in the techniques of modern cost-effective ECCE and PCI using the operating microscope. The wonderful success of the Tianjin Centre attests to Professor Yuan's eminent directorship and her steadfast commitment to combating mass cataract blindness in China

Adapted from the Asia-Pacific Journal of Ophthalmology, Vol. 11 No. 3, July 1999.

Brilliant Young Asian Ophthalmologists
of the 21st Century

The following young Asian ophthalmologists deserve special mention because they have distinguished themselves not only in ophthalmology, but also in fields outside of their academic disciplines. In the 21st Century, these multi-talented individuals are the ones who will lead ophthalmology towards a glorious future in Asia and around the world:

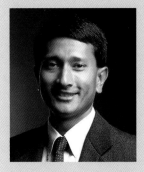

Medical Director, 39
Singapore National Eye
Centre (SNEC)
**Associate Professor
Vivian Balakrishnan**

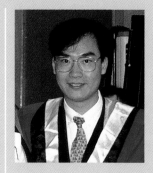

Chairman of the Department
of Ophthalmology, 40
Hong Kong University
Professor Dennis Lam

Associate Professor Vivian Balakrishnan, President's Scholar and Medical Director of SNEC, is one of the most brilliant minds in ophthalmology. Asides from his leadership role as the Medical Director of SNEC, he has also chaired and presented various social and health programmes on national television. From January to April 1996, he was the presenter for "Health Matters", a 13-episode Health Education series, and from August to September 1998, he was the chairman for "Heartware", a 6-episode series on national issues facing Singapore.

Professor Dennis Lam is the driving force behind the Department of Ophthalmology, Hong Kong University. That the local authorities chose him to spearhead ophthalmic developments in Hong Kong over Professor Mark Tso reflects their faith in the potential of brilliant young individuals to chart new frontiers for ophthalmology in the 21st Century. In 1996, Professor Lam was named one of the "Top Ten Outstanding Young Persons of the World".

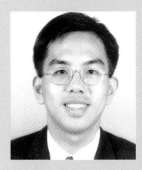

Assistant Professor, 31
National University
of Singapore; Registrar, SNEC
**Assistant Professor
Wong Tien Yin,
Singapore**

Assistant Professor Wong Tien Yin, President's Scholar, is no stranger to academic recognition and international accolades. He has won numerous awards for his contributions to national and international ophthalmology. In 1999, against other disciplines, he was voted one of the "Top Ten Most Outstanding Young Persons of the World". He is now in the United States pursuing a PhD at the prestigious Johns Hopkins Hospital.

Finally, a review of ophthalmic history — past, present and future —
by Associate Professor Chew Sek Jin (1998):

*"Three thousand years later, history repeats itself in Asia's unique contri-
butions to the management of yet another epidemic eye disorder. The dawn
of the new millennium again finds strong Asian leadership in international ophthalmic care. Myopia has now emerged as the commonest
ocular disorder worldwide and rises in incidence every year.*

*While affecting 25% of Caucasians, myopia is by far an Asian
problem — affecting up to 75% of some populations in this region. This
recent epidemic is ultimately linked to the shift from agrarian industries to
technologically dependent ones. Academic attainment and book learning
are needed to meet these demands. While a high regard for educational
attainment is a Confucian ethic, recent economic prosperity in Asia has
allowed high-quality public education to permeate all strata of society
and to dominate the lifestyles of every child and every family.*

*As with significant historical innovations in cataract surgery, the
roots of myopia management can similarly be traced to ancient China
where eye glasses were invented. In the 19th century, Europe took the lead
with empirical treatments using bifocal lenses, which were however
unsuccessful. In the last decade, investigators in the US brought news that
the retina regulates eye growth in myopia. Childhood myopia is thus an
adaptive ocular growth response to nearwork. The rapid neural and
ocular development in early life are most sensitive to changes in the visual
environment.*

*We are now at the threshold of rational, scientifically sound, and
effective myopia management strategies that can potentially benefit
millions of children around the globe. Where is this taking place? In Asia
of course. Institutions in Japan, Taiwan, China and Singapore now
lead in myopia epidemiology and randomized clinical trials. Singapore*

To all ophthalmologists from outside Asia, ...
 "Let us be united in our battle for quality ophthalmology." To everyone, I conclude: "What greater value than to use our skills to benefit mankind?"

is one of only four centres in the world vying for the elusive genes for this multifactorial disorder. Asian clinicians and scientists who have returned home from training in the top academic centres in the world are now taking ophthalmic research in their homelands to unforseen heights. As with the rebirth of the Asian cataract surgeon, the destiny of Asian ophthalmic research in the greatest eye problem in the world, rests as it should in Asian hands."

Conclusion

It is manifest that ophthalmology in Asia has awoken to a new dawn. To my Asian colleagues, I say: "The time has come for you to make significant contributions: deploy your skills for the promotion of quality eye-care in Asia."

To all ophthalmologists from outside Asia, I say: "Let us be united in our battle for quality ophthalmology."

To everyone, I conclude: "What greater value than to use our skills to benefit mankind?" ✳

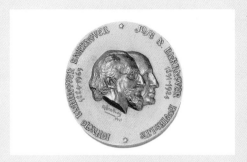

Barraquer Gold Medal Lecture
Towards Perfect Outcome in Cataract Surgery: The Eye Surgeon's Role

"In the 21st century, eye surgeons will play a critical role in cataract surgery. In their quest for the perfect outcome, not only must they improve their knowledge, polish their skills and enhance their surgical experiences, they must also exemplify the ethics of their profession."

Chapter 9

Towards Perfect Outcome in Cataract Surgery: The Eye Surgeon's Role

The Instituto Barraquer Gold Medal Lecture was delivered by the author at the 50th anniversary of the Barraquer Institute in Barcelona, Spain, on 8 June 1997. The Barraquer Institute, founded in 1947 by Professor Ignacio Barraquer (1884-1965), is the foremost institute of ophthalmology in Europe. The Barraquer family itself hails from an ancestry of four generations of ophthalmologists. The author felt deeply honoured to have been invited to deliver the lecture. He addressed an audience comprising of the leading lights of the ophthalmic world. In his lecture, the author highlighted the crucial role of eye surgeons in cataract surgery. He went on to underscore some characteristics of leading eye surgeons in the hope that this would motivate their contemporaries to perfection. Finally, he exhorted all professional ophthalmologists to be sensitive to patients' needs, and, at the same time, reminded them that ethical concerns would domi-nate the 21st century. The following is a reproduction of the original lecture, in slides.

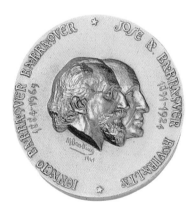

Medalla De Oro
Instituto Barraquer 1997:
Professor Arthur Lim
(Singapore)

TOWARDS PERFECT OUTCOME IN CATARACT SURGERY —THE EYE SURGEON'S ROLE

Professor Arthur Lim
Clinical Professor and Head
Department of Ophthalmology
National University of Singapore

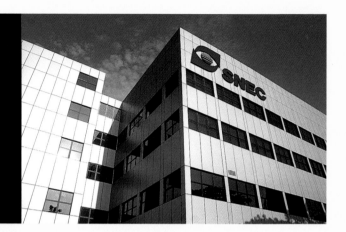

It is a great honour for me to deliver the 1997 Instituto Barraquer Gold Medal lecture at the 50th anniversary of the Barraquer Institute.

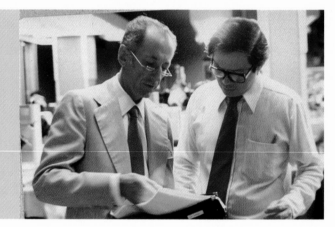

The Barraquers are an extraordinary family of five generations of ophthalmologists who have made outstanding contributions to world ophthalmology for decades.

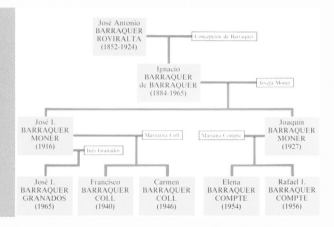

As I look at the events that contributed to quantum leaps in the quality and safety of ocular surgery, it is impossible not to encounter the great contributions the Barraquers have made in the half century of their clinic.

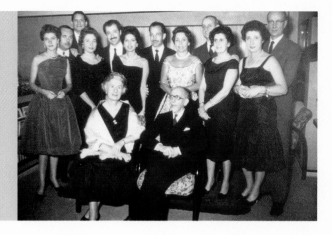

I emphasize two important points. First, in the 1950s, years before anyone else, the Barraquers used the microscope in surgery.

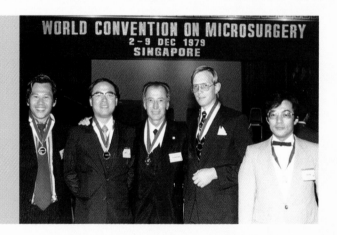

In 1947, 50 years ago, few eye surgeons were using the microscope. Thus the Barraquers achieved superior results in cataract surgery and in the surgery of other blinding conditions such as glaucoma, corneal eye diseases which require corneal transplantation and traumatic eye injuries.

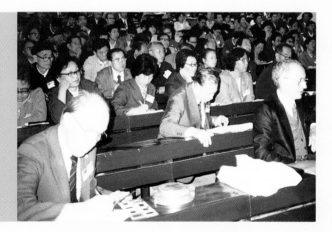

Second, the Barraquers were not selfish.

They generously taught quality and perfection throughout the world, including the developing world, in the tradition of the medical profession.

Much of the quality surgery in Asia — especially quality surgery under the mic roscope — have been due to the efforts of Joaquin Barraquer, strongly supported by his lovely wife Marianne.

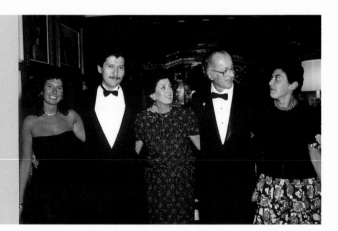

Joaquin, Asia will always remember your great contributions.

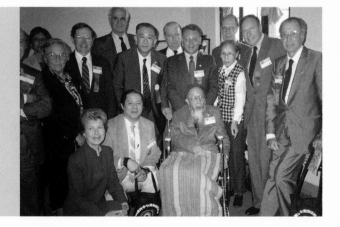

Professor Barraquer is universally admired and respected.

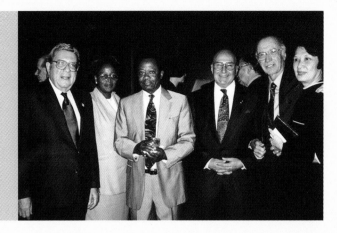

He is an honorary member of 26 national and foreign scientific associations. He has been invited as a special guest to over 40 meetings and has been awarded with 25 official Spanish as well as foreign decorations.

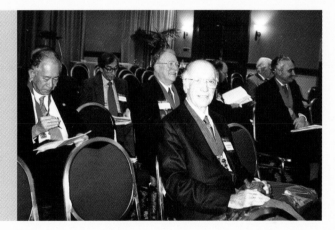

Why are top eye surgeons of the world, like the Barraquers, of growing importance in the 21st century?

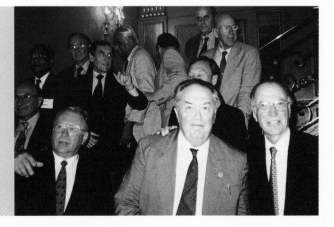

Because they are perfectionists. Not only do they innovate, but they also carefully and objectively evaluate every method and new technology they develop or use.

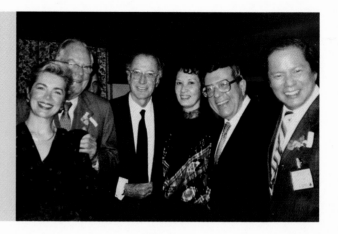

This contrasts with the worrying tendency to rush into new technology too rapidly, sometimes at the expense of patients.

Let me begin by giving the reason why I chose the topic "Towards Perfect Outcome In Cataract Surgery — the eye surgeon's role".

Cataract surgery is common and thousands of scientific papers are published each year. Why then should I produce another at this auspicious 50th anniversary?

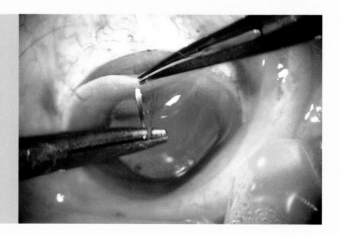

A quiet moment of reflection will reveal that quality cataract surgery is fascinating, for it embraces the personal attributes and qualities of thoughtful and caring surgeons, leaps in sophisticated technology, and the unceasing strife for surgical perfection. Yet, we have difficulties in even quantifying this outcome.

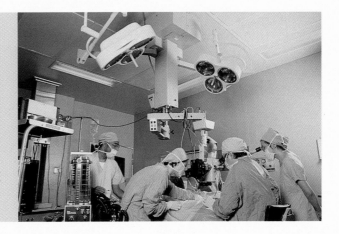

Cataract blindness contributes the lion's share of global blindness and causes 80% of blindness in some poor rural communities.

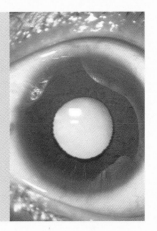

We are familiar with the difficulties and controversies in our attempts to introduce quality cataract surgery to the millions blind from cataract.

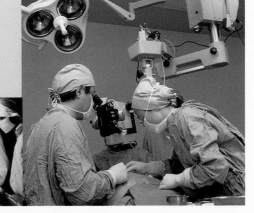

The forces of nature which have injured the human lens challenge us to find the ideal approach to mass cataract blindness. More important than this, we face another dilemma as concerns for human rights are raised — our ethics and our values must be scrutinized

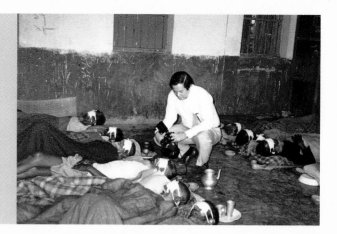

This has resulted in renewed concern for the patient's satisfaction after surgery.

These fascinating and important issues are personified by the Barraquers.

They have unceasingly in the past decades, challenged the problems of cataract surgery — clinically, surgically, academically, globally and ethically.

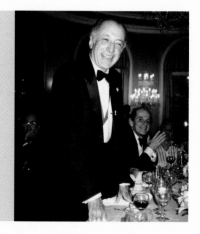

They continue to lead the world today and have already planned their contributions for tomorrow.

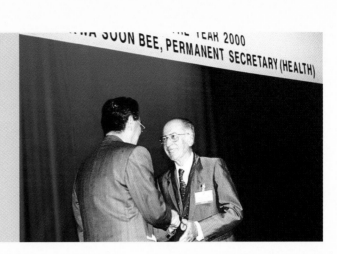

To achieve a perfect outcome, it is the surgeons and not the machines that are most important. It is Joaquin Barraquer and his family. It is they and not the numerous new machines.

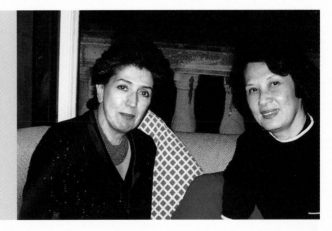

This address is not on machines, although they are important in modern eye surgery.

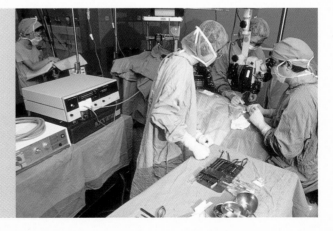

It is a reflection on the men behind the machines.

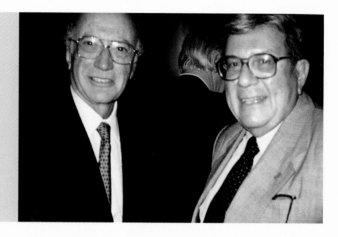

I am therefore not elaborating on the techniques and the details of phacoemulsification: the way to anaesthetise the eye, incision design, capsulorrhexis, hydrodissection, the alternative methods of phacoemulsification, the latest machines, the new viscoelastic materials, the best intraocular implants, sutureless closure of the wound and the alternatives in managing surgical complications in phacoemulsification.

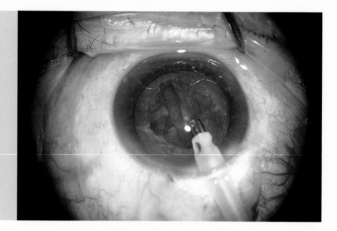

These are important but are already well documented in numerous scientific publications issued each year.

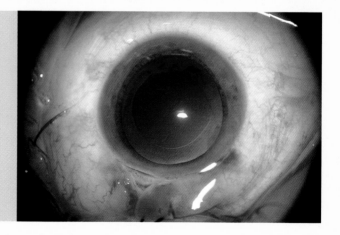

Perfection is a human attribute.

Our constant strife for perfect normal vision for our fellowmen is unmatched by machines whose lifetime and functions are limited, mindless and soulless.

I will address the issue of perfection in cataract surgery in the following five sections:
1. Worldwide demand for top eye surgeons
2. What is the perfect outcome?
3. How do we measure outcomes to reach for perfection?
4. Global trends in meeting our goals for perfection
5. Ethics and values in shaping the demand for surgical perfection

1. Worldwide Demand For Top Eye Surgeons

It is well known that economic growth of nations for decades was mainly based on manufacturing. More recently, the service industry has become important.

We have first to realise that different nations grow in different ways. While some would still depend on agriculture and others on manufacturing, a few countries are moving rapidly to develop their service and health industries.

The more economically advanced nations will move strongly towards health care service development. To achieve this, quality medical services have to be established.

One urgent move will be to recognize and retain the top eye surgeons who are known to achieve almost perfect results in their work.

In order to enable top talents to practise, these nations will change their medical registration rules. This has already happened in many countries including Europe.

What does this mean to us as individuals? How does all this affect eye surgeons? Why is it so important that we should talk about top talents?

To satisfy increasing patient's demand for quality service, nations will battle for top medical talent.

2 What Is The Perfect Outcome?
In the 21st century, the world will face challenges of affluence, advancing technology and the increasing demand for quality surgery.

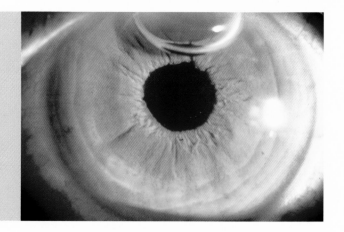

The educated patients will demand the best and they will seek perfect results from surgery.

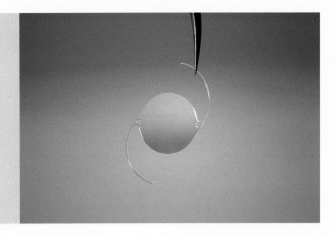

I emphasize that the surgeon who attains perfect results is one who does not ignore or hide his errors.

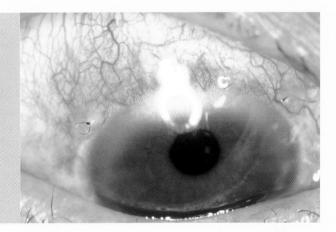

The wise surgeon would analyse, discuss and remember his errors for he knows that he can learn from them. This is invaluable to him and is fundamental for perfect surgery.

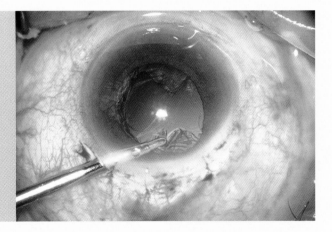

For perfect results, three factors are essential:
1. knowledge,
2. skill and
3. experience.

Knowledge

The surgeon must have in-depth understanding of the pathology of the condition he is managing. He needs sound knowledge of the surgical approach and the surgical problems that may arise.

He needs to critically and dispassionately appraise the latest scientific advances, and appreciate but not be a slave to world trends.

Knowledge is related to, but cannot be equated to, skill.

Skill

A skilled surgeon obtains perfect results, and is always gentle with tissues and pays meticulous attention to details.

Skill is a gift. It is a physical skill which is inherent, although with practice, the skill can be improved.

It can be illustrated by a tennis player. All the knowledge of tennis will not create a Michael Chiang.

The most important way to enhance surgical skill is through careful training as a resident.

The principles relating to skills were eloquently stated by the late Prof Yeoh Ghim Seng, the first local Professor of Surgery of Singapore:
"... all surgical trainees must not be allowed to operate on patients during their early stages of postgraduate surgical education. They must be shown how to do things properly so that they will, under proper guidance, become safe surgeons."

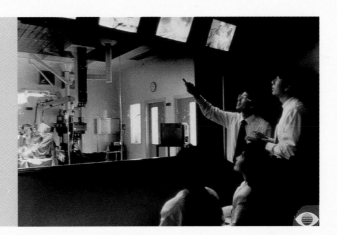

Experience
Experience does not mean that the surgeon must be old.

Experience means that the surgeon should observe, assist and perform surgery himself, initially with assistance, and later on his own.

Experience means that he has to learn every procedure carefully, step by step, especially the complicated procedures, to attain perfect results.

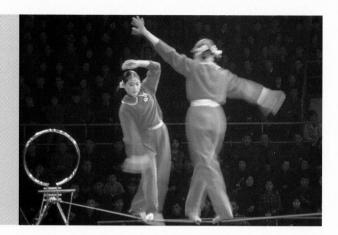

Experience would mean that a surgeon would need to follow a good surgeon, and follow him through 10, 50, or 100 procedures.

The identification of a first rate surgeon is essential. Young doctors will learn his good habits and techniques, why he has few complications and why his results are almost perfect.

This is the only way to ensure that surgeons of the future will be just as good and hopefully even better.

It is well known that an hour with a skilled and wise master surgeon is worth a month of study.

On the other hand, if surgeons follow a second rate surgeon, they will end up as third rate surgeons.

Unfortunately, some young surgeons think that as soon as they have seen or assisted in a surgical procedure once or twice, they can perform the operation effectively. This can be disastrous.

I was distressed when a young ophthalmologist said to me, "How can I learn new techniques if I do not practise on my patients?" And I replied, "Practise? On the eyes of your patients? Why don't you use the laboratory?" And the answer was, "But that's not the same. Anyway, the 'learning curve' is accepted around the world!"

Surgeons must remember that the patients' interest is foremost and that first, do no harm, especially in a new surgical procedure.

3. How Do We Measure Outcomes To Reach For Perfection?

Can we measure excellence and perfect outcome?

The surgical skill of a doctor can be difficult to assess. However, for certain operations in some specialties, measurement of excellence is easier.

For example in ophthalmology, operations such as cataract extraction can be measured by the visual results and we know that a good surgeon can restore normal vision (20/40) in almost 100% of patients.

More exacting outcomes of $^{20}/_{30}$ or $^{20}/_{20}$ or "assessment of subjective visual function" will be used more widely in the future.

The skills of eye surgeons have been evaluated in several countries. In the USA, the American Board of Eye Surgery was formed on 20 July 1985.

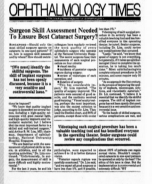

In the 21st century, I predict that more and more surgeons from all over the world will voluntarily be asking for their skills to be evaluated.

"Should only the most skilled surgeons operate on one-eye patients? If so, how is a surgeon's skill assessed, and by whom? How should restrictions be imposed?"

I decided to base my assessment of each cataract operation on three criteria: visual results, incidence of posterior capsule rupture during surgery, and surgical review of videotapes of operations with complications.

As expected, this had considerable impact. The quality of surgery improved; the patients were assured of good visual results; and the residents received good training.

Videotaping of every operation in its entirety has been invaluable and was effective for teaching, benefiting everyone in the operating theatre.

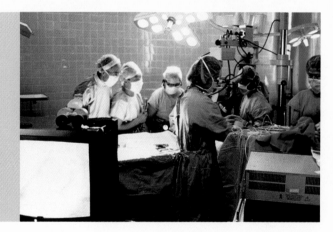

I am making a prediction of the way surgery will move in one decade. It is rather controversial today but all good surgeons have to prepare for it.

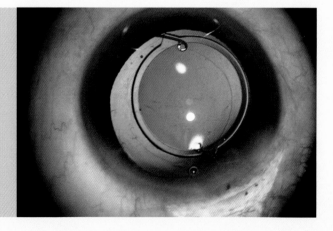

The controversy of giving a videotape of surgery to patients is likely to become a standard practice.

If we look at other professionals, the lawyers have to appear in court with every word being recorded and now televised; the architects and engineers have to present and sign their plans on paper — their clients and peers can identify from these records who are excellent.

4. Global Trends In Meeting Our Goals For Perfection

Phacoemulsification is an elegant high-technology operation and is the operation of choice for cataract in the USA.

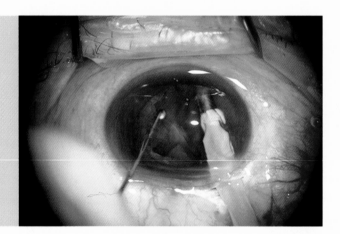

The small incision allows rapid post-operative visual improvement with less astigmatism and achieves greater patient satisfaction. Thus, in the wealthier nations, the procedure has become popular.

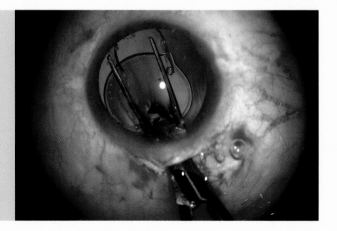

The world has entered a fascinating period and new surgical approaches are introduced each month, making it difficult for many surgeons to keep up.

Innovators are never satisfied and continue to search for safer surgery with better outcome.

The use of the YAG laser and the use of electromagnetic forces to disintegrate the nucleus and the experiments with small incision of the anterior capsule so that soft material can be injected into the lens capsule to achieve accommodation are exciting developments.

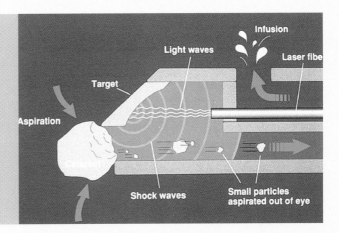

In addition to ensuring detailed steps to prevent endophthalmitis, complications which can arise with anaesthesia from retrobulbar or peribulbar injection can be prevented by using eyedrops and subconjunctival local anaesthesia instead.

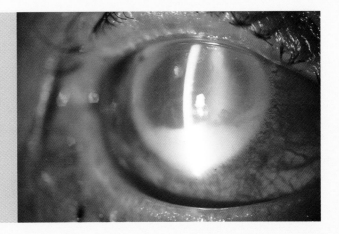

The anterior capsule opening with capsulorrhexis, although it does not give superior results, ensures that the implant will be in-the-bag. If small enough, 1mm in the periphery of the anterior capsule, a soft or liquid implant becomes a possibility.

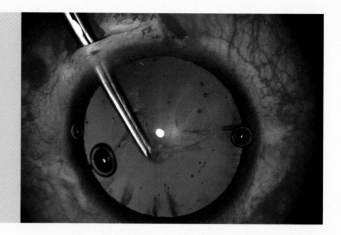

The nucleus disintegration with phacoemulsification may be replaced by other methods such as the use of the YAG laser or electromagnetic forces. A soft or liquid implant has attracted many enthusiasts hoping to restore accommodation to the eye.

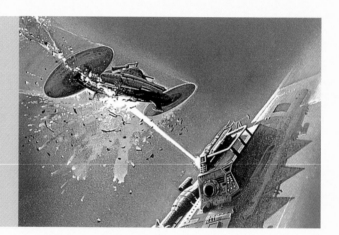

The Latest May Not Be The Best
Over the past few decades, surgical progress has moved forward as a result of innovative technological advances. It is always fashionable to have the latest equipment and to be performing the newest techniques.

A surgeon must always question whether the latest surgery being evaluated is the best. It may be prudent to ask, "Are there situations when the latest is not the best?"

In recent years, health costs have become a major issue, not only for developing countries, but also for developed nations. Even the wealthiest country in the world, the United States of America, has decided to intervene.

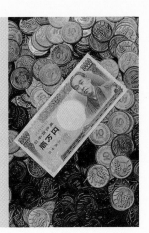

All governments and eye surgeons, particularly those from the less wealthy countries, have the grave responsibility of deciding on the suitability of an innovation — as sometimes, the latest may not be the best.

ASIA — Wealth And Its Contrast
Is it possible to introduce quality cataract and implant surgery in Asia? What are the problems?

Cataract is a massive problem in Asia, accounting for more than 50% to 80% of blindness. This has caused misery and socio-economic agony to unoperated patients now estimated to be well over 10 million.

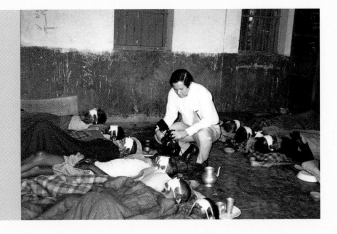

Koh (1995) at the Arthur and Frank Payne Lecture at Stanford University reported that in the past few years, the world has experienced a change of historic importance. East Asia has risen in the world economy.

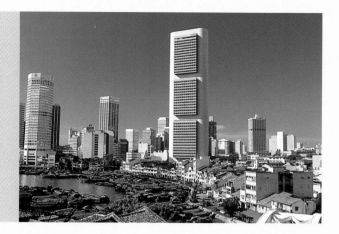

In Purchasing Power Parity (PPP) terms, East Asia's GDP was already larger than that of either the United States or the European Union, and by 2005 would be bigger than both combined.

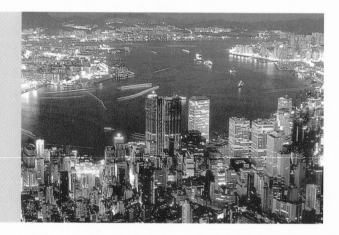

The Contrast In Wealth

Table 1		
Country	Per Capita GNP (1993)	GDP per head (1996 forecasts)
Japan	US$31,490	US$40,500
Singapore	US$19,850	US$30,301
USA	-	US$28,440
Hong Kong	US$18,060	US$27,040
France	-	US$27,000
Italy	-	US$20,670
United Kingdom	-	US$20,490
Ausulia	US$17,500	US$20,200
New Zealand	US$12,600	US$17,230
Taiwan	US$10,852	US$14,470
Spain	-	US$13,930
South Korea	US$ 7,660	US$11,580
Malaysia	US$ 3,140	US$ 4,261
Thailand	US$ 2,110	US$ 3,110
China	US$ 490	US$ 520
India	US$ 300	US$ 335
Nepal	US$ 190	-
Bangladesh	US$ 220	-

Source: Far East Economic Review Asia 1996 Yearbook
The Economist - The World In 1996

Barraquer Lecture 1997

It was hard for many people in Europe and America to comprehend the reality that East Asia is today the new growth locomotive for the world economy.

The rise of East Asia in the world economy has either escaped the attention of many people in the West or has been greeted with disbelief because it has been so rapid and so unexpected.

The infant mortality rate of the United States (8.3) is higher than those of Japan (4.4), Singapore (5.0), Taiwan (5.7) and Hong Kong (6.4), showing that quality public health has already been established in Asia and that the goals for perfection in cataract surgery will follow.

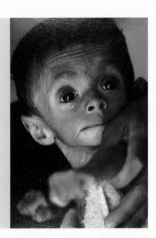

Tianjin — A Model For Quality Cataract Surgery

The Tianjin International Intraocular Implant Training Centre, an influential model for quality cataract surgery in developing countries, was opened on 29 September 1989.

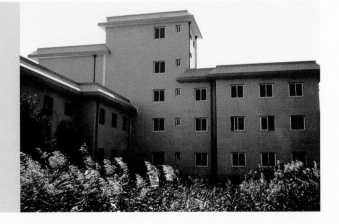

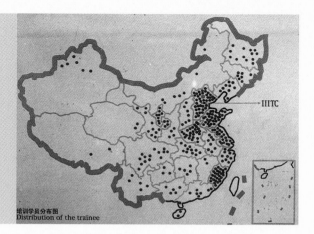

This Centre has trained 2,000 ophthalmologists from around China. It has organised 34 courses (19 in the centre, 15 outside the centre) in implant microsurgery for ophthalmologists from different provinces of China.

培训学员分布图
Distribution of the trainee

5. Ethics And Values In Shaping The Demand For Surgical Perfection

For some years, excellent surgeons have been accused, quite correctly, to be too concerned with high technology, new surgical approaches, expensive new lasers and ultrasounds, but have ignored the ethics of a good surgeon.

Strength of Character
An essential factor for excellence is the strength of character of top surgeons. Competitiveness is vital.

Different people see differently when they look out of the window. Some see the stars and some see the mud. Those who only see the mud will never excel.

In the past decades, I noticed characteristics of surgeons who seek perfection.

They are:

1. They associate with other top surgeons or leading professionals and outstanding people outside their professional circles. This association is a vital continuing process of learning from leading minds.

2. They identify the key issues quickly and they always think hardest about issues which matter most. For example, in cataract surgery, the single most important complication which can cause blindness is endophthalmitis.

In risky situations, good surgeons will only act after most careful and long deliberations.

Top surgeons spend much time teaching their colleagues. Teaching has always been a hallmark of the truly great surgeon and they must not be insecure and view younger colleagues as potential rivals.

Instead, surgeons must prepare their younger colleagues to hopefully surpass them in the future, for that is the basis for progress.

Good surgeons are always inventive, always thinking how to improve themselves.

Good surgeons must adapt to circumstances, especially when they operate in different hospitals and different countries. Hospitals have their own equipment and limitations.

There are many other characteristics of leading surgeons. They are sensible, cautious, prudent and discreet. To attain perfection, goodness and virtue are essential.

Good surgeons must think of ethics and values, for surgeons are only of value if they use their skills for the benefit of their fellowmen.

Patients' Desire Versus Medical Scientific Advances

It is well known that the practice of medicine has changed from the art of medicine to the science of medicine.

But patients are beginning to resist scientific medicine and in some countries, patients exert their rights to make their own decisions.

This had led to the assumption that what is right for the treatment of the disease must also be right for the patient. It may be said that this had led to excellent management of the patient's disease but bad management of the patient.

A perfect operation cannot be achieved without considering the needs of the patient. Good surgeons must learn this — even if it conflicts with the scientific management of the disease.

Conclusion

The 21st century will bring fascinating progress in all areas of life. Patients' expectation for surgical perfection will increase and eye surgeons must meet this demand.

Almost 100% visual outcome can be achieved by eye surgeons who have mastered cataract surgery, for it is the surgeon's ability and not the constantly changing technology that is essential for success.

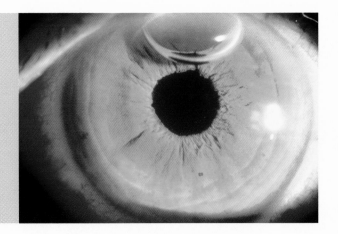

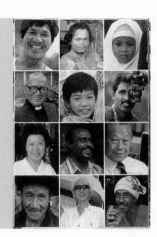

I emphasize that successful cataract surgeons with perfect results have three basic attributes — knowledge, skill and experience. In addition, wise surgeons will not ignore the patients' desires and hopes which after all are what clinical practice is all about.

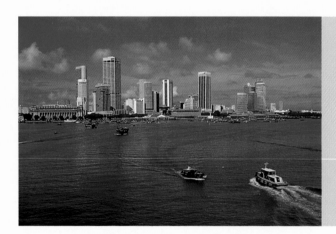

The End

AMERICAN JOURNAL OF OPHTHALMOLOGY®

JUNE 1999
VOLUME 123

EDITORIAL

The Dilemma of Ophthalmic Changes Spreads to Asia

ARTHUR S. M. LIM, MBBS, FRCS

Chapter 10

EDITORIAL

AMERICAN JOURNAL OF OPHTHALMOLOGY, JUNE 1999

The Dilemma of Ophthalmic Changes Spreads to Asia

———————

"I WANT GOOD VISION" will be the cry of everyone, everywhere in the next millennium. The note a Hindu patient wrote to me recently is a dramatic reaction of a blind patient whose vision was restored: "God gave me vision and nature took it away. You have restored my vision — to me you are God."

Good vision is important throughout life. As age advances and physical agility decreases, the enjoyment of life becomes increasingly visual — to many, it is reading; to others, it is television. To a steadily growing number, good vision is required for the use of modern electronic devices, computers and information technology equipment.

In the nineteenth century, cost was not a problem when eye doctors could only offer their patients palliative and consoling words. The twentieth century brought high technology and increases in health care costs.

Good vision is important throughout life. As age advances and physical agility decreases, the enjoyment of life becomes increasingly visual... .

Reprinted from the American Journal of Ophthalmology, Vol. 123, Arthur S.M. Lim, The Dilemma of Ophthalmic Changes Spreads to Asia, 715-716, 1999, with permission from Elsevier Science.

After World War II, great advances were made. This period has been considered the glorious years of ophthalmology... .

When a person is well, he or she may question health care costs, but when a person is dying, in pain, or in danger of losing vision, that person will pray and fight for the best, and cost will not matter.

After World War II, great advances were made. This period has been considered the glorious years of ophthalmology, when it was supported with great enthusiasm and ocular surgeons throughout the world were admired. The discovery of penicillin, followed by the introduction of numerous antibiotics, prevented blindness from trachoma, corneal ulcer, and other infections. Ocular surgery was performed with precision under the operating microscope; microinstruments and microsutures and cataract surgery advanced dramatically with extracapsular cataract extraction and posterior chamber intraocular lenses. Additionally, laser technology, ultrasonography, computerized perimetry and biochemical materials advanced ophthalmology.

Modern mass communications informed everyone, everywhere about the wonders of modern ophthalmology, and public demand for quality eye care escalated. When a person is well, he or she may question health care costs, but when a person is dying, in pain, or in danger of losing vision, that person will pray and fight for the best, and cost will not matter. This contradiction was eloquently summarized by a former British Minister for Health, Enoch Powell, "There is virtually no limit to the amount of health care an individual is capable of absorbing."[1]

There is no escape from the "trillion-dollar health crisis", as high costs, high technology, and the increasing number of patients demanding quality care can lead us in only one direction — an explosion of health care costs in the next millennium. This is a major dilemma affecting governments, corporations in the health enterprise, physicians and patients. Major changes in eye care will be necessary in the next millennium. It is wise to discuss these openly even if some are unpleasant and generate controversy. How can we progress if we fear discussion of important changes for a better tomorrow?[2]

In recent years, dramatic medical progress has been complicated

by serious public concern; these are the years of contradiction. The primary cause of public concern is the escalating expense of medical care, which has resulted in health care costs reaching 10% of gross national product in some countries and up to 15% of the gross national product in the United States.

Governments and corporations have acted to control increases in health care costs by reforming medical services. Unfortunately, these reforms tend to treat patients as statistics, overlooking the fact that every patient suffers the misery of illness alone.

Health reforms will need to focus on costs while striving to maintain quality. Preventing unnecessary expenditure is essential, but this is quite different from cutting costs without reason, which will lower the quality of care. Many issues are sensitive, and decisions require a delicate balance. Inappropriate cost control can easily become an obstacle to progress. When issues are complex, we should remind ourselves of what Asia's celebrated Nobel laureate, Rabindranath Tagore said, "If you are not open, the door to the truth will be shut."

The journey in search of quality eye care and good vision in the more developed nations is difficult. Asian nations are experiencing similar difficulties, made worse by the influence of diverse cultures, races, religions, and climates and by financial limitations.

Is quality eye care and good vision for the population of Asia possible? Asia is a region of fascinating contrasts, with more than half the world's population and more than half the world's blindness. Governments and health care corporations are making heroic efforts to establish quality eye care services throughout Asia.

Ophthalmic training institutions are improving programs, for example, video conferencing between eye centers is disseminating information rapidly. When this is combined with clinical audits and outcome

Inappropriate cost control can easily become an obstacle to progress.

The journey in search of quality eye care and good vision in the more developed nations is difficult. Asian nations are experiencing similar difficulties, made worse by the influence of diverse cultures, races, religions, and climates and by financial limitations.

evaluations, high standards will spread quickly. Numerous ophthalmic centres of excellence will be established throughout Asia, and ophthalmologists from developed nations will have the exciting opportunity to help ophthalmologists provide quality eye care to the people of Asia.

Alvin Toffler, a celebrated American futurist, has argued that where knowledge is critical, the highly intelligent and specialised professionals will demand empowerment and the ability to determine their own development[3]. Ophthalmologists need to validate this forecast by working together, working efficiently and promoting quality eye care services.

For decades, the wonders of modern ophthalmology were limited to the cities, but recently, rapid economic growth has gradually spread information throughout rural Asia. Even in remote mountain and desert areas, more victims of eye disease are crying out, "I want good vision!" With the participation of government, the World Health Organization (WHO), the World Bank, non-governmental organizations, and with professional leadership by ophthalmologists, we have an opportunity to advance ophthalmic care throughout Asia. The next millennium will be fascinating when the joy of vision spreads and everyone can embrace the wonders of modern ophthalmology.

Ocular surgeons who are not fortunate enough to have worked in rural Asia, where the neglected blind are burdened with poverty, ignorance, and misery, need to sit back and quietly reexamine the principles that elevated our profession to one of honour and high esteem. Each of us needs to ask: What have I done in my life — have I used my skill to restore vision to the millions blinded from cataracts and used my talents to aid the millions afflicted with other vision-threatening diseases?

For us as ophthalmologists, there can be no greater value than to use our professional skills to ensure good vision for the people of the world. ✳

Ocular surgeons... need to sit back and quietly reexamine the principles that elevated our profession to one of honour and high esteem.

Chapter 11

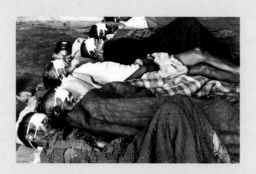

WORLDEYES

"The 20th century has drawn to a close, leaving behind countless victims of eye disease. The World Eye Surgeons Society, a uniquely Asian initiative, is committed to bringing relief to the millions suffering from blindness in Asia and other developing countries."

Charity Wai
Secretary-General, World Eye Surgeons Society
Chief Operating Officer, Singapore National Eye Centre

Chapter 10

AMERICAN JOURNAL OF OPHTHALMOLOGY®

JUNE 1999 • VOLUME 127

INDEX ISSUE

AJO®

MONTHLY SINCE 1884

Visit our Web Site and Authors Interactive® at http://www.ajo.com/

ELSEVIER
ISSN 0002-9394

The Dilemma of Ophthalmic Changes Spreads to Asia

Editorial
American Journal of Ophthalmology,
June 1999

Chapter 11

WORLDEYES

———

"The 20th century has drawn to a close, leaving behind countless victims of eye disease."

Everywhere in Asia, even in the remote mountain and desert areas, more and more victims with vision impaired by eye disease are crying, "I want to see." The World Health Organization (WHO) and non-government organizations (NGOs) have stepped in, despite occasional disagreements in approach, to succour the victims of eye disease.

A group of eye surgeons who are based in Singapore together with their co-workers, foresaw the increasing importance of eye surgeons. For it had become clear that while blindness from infection and malnutrition had rapidly come under control, blindness from eye diseases requiring the care of qualified eye surgeons was on the increase.

This is the scenario against which the World Cataract Surgeons Society (WORLDCATS) was formed. WORLDCATS, mooted at the Singapore National Eye Centre's (SNEC) first international meeting in 1993, was registered on June 3, 1994. It was proposed as an international movement of eye surgeons dedicated to the control of mass cataract blindness in developing countries, and especially in Asia, where millions are blind from the condition.

More support would be needed to control cataract blindness and other causes of blindness like glaucoma and diabetic retinopathy. In fact, glaucoma will be the world's leading cause of blindness and will pose a major challenge to eye surgeons in 10 years.

Singapore-based, WORLDCATS began to implement various activities in phases with the objectives to 1) promote opportunities for training and skills transfer in cataract eye surgery to ophthalmologists in developing countries; 2) promote quality assurance in eye surgery world-wide; and 3) achieve an initial target of performing 1,000,000 cataract implant operations through the united efforts of volunteer eye surgeons. These activities stimulated the interest of over 1,000 eye surgeons and volunteers from 94 countries world-wide, and this number will grow in time. In addition, its links with eye centres throughout the world will also be expanded. With the spread of interest beyond cataract, the society's name has been updated to encompass other eye diseases and surgery like glaucoma, diabetic retinopathy, and corneal transplantation. Hence the new name — World Eye Surgeons Society (WORLDEYES) has been adopted. But good labels do not fade away easily, and the inaugural name WORLDCATS still fits comfortably whenever the organization is mentioned.

Unique Model — International Intraocular Implant Training Centre, Tianjin, People's Republic of China

The International Intraocular Implant Training Centre (IIITC) was opened in Tianjin on September 29, 1989, after much discussion between Professor Arthur Lim, Founding President of WORLDEYES and the ophthalmologists and government officials in Tianjin. Under the sterling leadership of Prof Yuan Jia-Qin, the IIITC has achieved spectacular results and is recognised as a successful model for mass cataract control programmes for China and other developing nations. The Centre has performed more than 120,000 cases of quality implant surgery with its network of 16 affiliated hospitals, and aims to restore normal vision to 1,000,000 blind victims.

Further Expansion

At the IIITC's 10th Anniversary celebrations in September 1999, the existing Memorandum of Understanding between the Tianjin International Intraocular Implant Training Centre (IIITC) — now renamed the Tianjin Medical University Eye Centre (TMUEC) — and the SNEC was expanded by Associate Professor Vivian Balakrishnan and Dr Sun Hui-Min, second echelon leaders of the two centres.

Following the glowing success of the Tianjin Centre, four other centres have been established in succession:

Xiamen Eye Centre

The Xiamen Eye Centre (XEC) was officially opened on November 8,

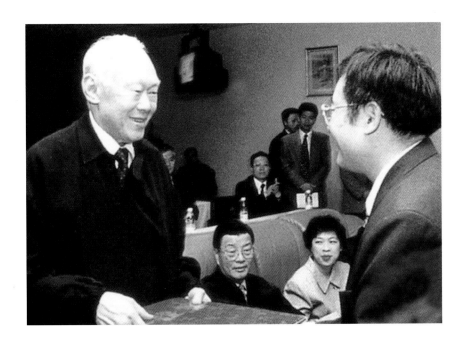

A/P Vivian Balakrishnan, SNEC's Medical Director, exchanging plagues with IIITC's Director, Prof Sun Hui-Min, to expand ties between SNEC and IIITC as sister centres.

Professor Hong Rong-Zhao presented the Research & Training Memorandum of Understanding to Singapore's Senior Minister Lee Kuan Yew during the latter's visit to China on 8 December 1997.

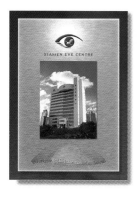

Brochure of Xiamen Eye Centre.

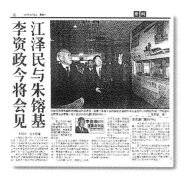

S'pore helps set up fifth eye centre in China with focus on training

SINGAPORE has helped set up yet another eye centre in China, the Xiamen Eye Centre.

The 14-storey building, which has outpatient, inpatient and teaching facilities, was built at a cost of $7 million and will be opened officially on Nov 14.

The Singapore Eye Foundation donated US$280,000 (S$434,000) towards building the centre, and the Singapore National Eye Centre (Snec) contributed equipment of the same value to the Xiamen centre.

Snec's medical director, Professor Arthur Lim, also made personal donations of about $250,000 to the centre. The rest of the money came from the Chinese government and other private donors.

This is the fifth centre that the Snec has helped develop in China. The others are the International Intraocular Implant Training Centre in Tianjin, the Jinan World Cataract Centre in Shandong and two eye centres in Yinchuan and Ningxia, in Northern China.

At a press conference yesterday, Prof Lim said that the

main focus of the Xiamen centre will be training.

He said that although the centre will be able to treat some 100,000 outpatients and 4,000 warded patients a year, there are hopes to train many ophthalmologists in cataract surgery to help treat cataracts, which is China's biggest eye problem. The others are glaucoma and short-sightedness.

Doctors and officials from Xiamen have been at the Snec this week to tie up more joint projects between the two centres.

For example, both centres have agreed to conduct a joint study into the severity and extent of short-sightedness in Xiamen.

Also in the pipeline are training programmes in the treatment of major blinding conditions such as glaucoma, and the formation of a group of top international eye surgeons, who will use Singapore as a base to extend assistance to developing countries in Asia.

Prof Lim said that the Snec is ready to bring more eye centres to other parts of Asia like India, Myanmar and Vietnam.

Press report on Xiamen Eye Centre,
The Straits Times, Saturday,
25 October 1997.

Press report on visit to Xiamen Eye Centre
by Senior Minister Lee Kuan Yew, Lianhe
Zaobao, Singapore Chinese Press, Monday,
8 December 1997.

1997 in the People's Republic of China as a variation and extension of the Tianjin Centre model.

Under the outstanding and tireless efforts of its Founding Medical Director, Prof Hong Rong-Zhou, the Xiamen Eye Centre has been transformed from a poorly equipped medical institution to a purpose-built, well-equipped eye centre in southern China. Housed in a 15-storey building with a total floor area of 15,000 m², the Centre's facilities include outpatient clinics, five major operating theatres equipped with audio-visual laser rooms, microsurgery wet labs, 180-bed inpatient eye wards, and research laboratories. The Centre currently serves 100,000 outpatients, 2,500 inpatients and 3,200 major surgeries annually.

Major Centre of Influence

Xiamen Eye Centre has become the key training centre from where ophthalmic knowledge and skills are spread countrywide. Since its open-

SM Lee Meets Premier Jiang Zeming and Zhu Rongji

Senior Minister Lee Kuan Yew visited the Xiamen Eye Centre before he ended his interview in Xiamen, China, yesterday. The eye centre, a 15-storey tall building which accommodates 180 beds, was built with an investment of over S$1.8 million dollars. The establishment of this eye centre was proposed and developed by Professor Arthur Lim Siew Ming, medical director of the Singapore National Eye Centre and Professor Hong Rong Zhao, medical director of the Xiamen Eye Centre. The Xiamen Eye Centre was officially opened on 8 November 1997.

The Xiamen Eye Centre and Singapore National Eye Centre have developed a series of programmes to encourage the cooperation and exchange of medical skills and technology between both centres. Now, both centres can exchange information on the condition of eye patients and treatment over the internet.

Abridged translation
Lianhe Zaobao, Singapore Chinese Press
8 December 1997, Monday

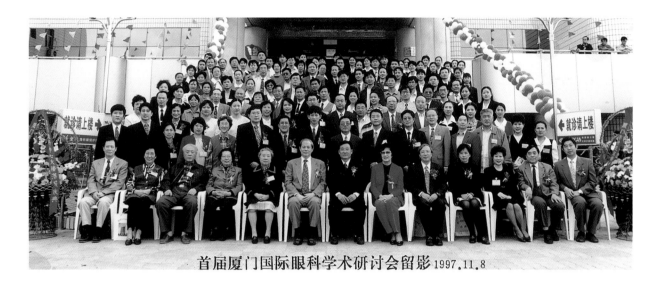

首届厦门国际眼科学术研讨会留影1997.11.8

*Opening ceremony of Xiamen Eye Centre,
8 November 1997.*

ing in November 1997, the Centre has embarked on numerous training programmes both locally and internationally. With the assistance of Professor Arthur Lim, Xiamen Eye Centre has successfully organised three large scale training workshops in ECCE and Phacoemulsification. It has also hosted an international meeting and co-organised several major ophthalmic conferences in China.

The Xiamen Eye Centre will continue to influence ophthalmology nationally and internationally.

Cataract Surgery Training Centre of Jinan, Shandong Province

Jinan, the capital of populous Shandong province with 80 million people, is home to the Cataract Surgery Training Centre of the Jinan Municipal Central Hospital. Prof Chen Wei, with her dedicated team, has been performing quality cataract surgery as well as training eye surgeons. Occupying a two-storey building, the Centre started its services in April 1996 with the bulk of surgical instruments purchased with a generous private donation from Prof Arthur Lim, President of WORLDEYES. Prof Lim officially opened the Centre on September 24, 1996.

In May 1997, the First Shandong Province Cataract Implant Training and Phacoemulsification Course was organised. The occasion was graced by top officials of the Shandong province and the Jinan Municipal Central Hospital administration. A pioneering team of ophthalmologists from the Singapore National Eye Centre, consisting of Drs Ang Chong Lye, Esther Fu and Wee Tze Lin demonstrated cataract surgeries ranging from low-cost ECCE technique, using only air for lens implantation, to state-of-the-art small incision phacoemulsification with insertion of foldable intraocular lens to an audience of over 100 delegates.

Department of Ophthalmology, People's Hospital, Ningxia
Department of Ophthalmology, 2nd Affiliated Hospital of Lanzhou Medical College

These two centres represented WORLDEYES' moves to set up units to serve the inner regions of China. Ningxia and Lanzhou are both situated in northwest China. The province of Ningxia, approximately 1,000 km from Beijing, has a population of 5 million people. It is an autonomous region with a large community of Muslims. In July 1996, eye surgeons from WORLDEYES visited the department to determine the feasibility of developing it into a training base unit to serve those living in the remote regions. The Centre handles about 25,000 outpatient visits each year.

Lanzhou, the capital of Gansu province in northwest China, has the reputation of being the city where the fabled silk road originated. Gansu province has a population of 27 million while the capital city Lanzhou supports 3.5 million people. It is now a major industrial area for China, providing petrochemical products and nuclear power. The 2nd Affiliated Hospital of Lanzhou Medical College is a general hospital with 750 beds. The Department of Ophthalmology has 10 eye doctors assisted by a team of eye-care professionals and support staff.

These two units will play a useful role in outreach programmes to serve the victims of blindness in the remote and rural areas of China.

Affiliated Centre: Zhongshan Ophthalmic Centre, Guangzhou

The Zhongshan Ophthalmic Centre (ZOC) of Sun Yat-sen University of Medical Sciences is located in Guangzhou. The Centre was founded by the late famous ophthalmic specialists, Professors YaoZhen (Eugene) Chan and Wenshu (Winifred) Mao. It was the first modern ophthalmic centre in China to integrate eye-care, teaching, eye research and blindness prevention activities in one setting.

Prof Lim, President, World Eye Surgeons Society recently renewed his longstanding ties with the Centre which started since the time of Professors Eugene Chen and Winifred Mao some 20 years ago. He will deliver the Winifred Mao Memorial Lecture — "The Challenges and Reforms in the 21st Century" — at the 12th Afro-Asian Congress of Ophthalmology International Meeting, Guangzhou, 11-14 November 2000.

The Centre will continue to collaborate closely with WORLDEYES in the fight against blindness from cataract and other major blinding conditions.

The Future

With the common vision of "Spreading Light Across the World" and the growing number of over 1,000 members and volunteers from 94 countries around the globe, the WORLDEYES movement will march confidently forward into the 21st Century, promulgating new knowledge and techniques, stimulating development, emphasizing quality eye surgery to restore vision and to bring relief to the millions of blind victims in the world. ✳

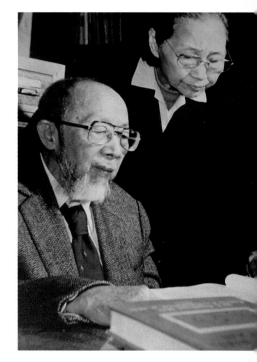

Professor Eugene Chan with his wife, Professor Winifred Mao

ACTIVITIES OF WORLDEYES VOLUNTEERS IN THE PEOPLE'S REPUBLIC OF CHINA

20 - 21 May 1995	Surgery course, Jinan Central Municipal Hospital, Jinan, Shandong Province.
24 September 1995	Free mass eye-screening, Tianjin.
23 - 29 September 1995	Teaching course and live surgery demonstrations, IIITC, Tianjin.
19 - 24 July 1996	Visit to Ningxia People's Hospital, Yinchuan Province.
20 - 22 September 1996	1st WORLDCATS international meeting and 2nd IIITC meeting, Tianjin.
6 - 11 November 1996	1st conjoint teaching course cum live surgery demonstration, Xiamen Eye Centre.
16 - 19 May 1997	Scientific meeting and training course, IIITC.
20 - 21 May 1997	1st Shandong Province phacoemulsification and cataract implant training course, Jinan, Shandong Province.
3 - 5 March 1998	Participated at the WHO / Ministry of Health / International NGDO Second Coordination Meeting for the Prevention of Blindness in China, Beijing.
10 - 15 September 1999	IIITC 10th Anniversary celebrations: conjoint 13th ICIMRK, 2nd World Eyes International Meeting and 4th IIITC International Meeting.
21 - 23 April 2000	Joint organiser of "This Century's Challenges", in association with Parkway Group Healthcare Pte Ltd, Parkway Healthcare Foundation and the Singapore National Eye Centre.
2 - 4 December 2000	Joint organiser of the 4th Singapore National Eye Centre International Meeting and 3rd World Eye Surgeons Society International Meeting in commemoration of Singapore National Eye Centre's 10th Anniversary. The World Eye Surgeons Society Meeting will also see the inauguration of the "Sir John Wilson Lecture", created in memory of the gallant man who fought to free the world from needless blindness.

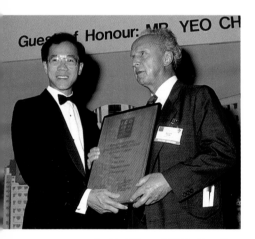

Sir John Wilson with Mr Yeo Cheow Tong,
Minister for Health, Singapore

The following awards were presented to various institutions and individuals for their significant contribution to the fight against mass cataract blindness and for their promotion of cataract surgery with intraocular implants.

WORLDEYES INSTITUTIONAL AWARDS

1999

- 120,000   Tianjin Medical University Eye Centre (formerly known as International Intraocular Implant Training Centre)
- 20,000   Xiamen Eye Centre
- 12,000   Cataract Surgery Centre of Jinan Municipal Centre Hospital
- 8,000   Zhongshan Ophthalmic Centre
- 2,000   Department of Ophthalmology, Ningxia People's Hospital
- 2,000   Eye Department, 2nd Affiliated Hospital, Lanzhou Medical College

WORLDEYES INDIVIDUAL AWARDS

1995

- **Certificate of Achievement**   Dr Chen Wei *Shangdong, PRC*
  (1,000 and above cataracts and IOLs)   Dr Reggie Seimon *Sri Lanka*

1996

- **WORLDCATS Gold Medal**   Prof Yuan Jia-Qin *Tianjin, PRC*

- **Distinguished Achievement Award**   Prof Yuan Jia-Qin *Tianjin, PRC*
  (5,000 and above cataracts and IOLs)

- **Special Achievement Award**   Dr G Venkataswamy *Aravind Centre, India*

- **Distinguished Award**   IMPACT

- **Certificate of Achievement**   Dr Huang Xiao-Yan *Tangshan Hebei, PRC*
  (1,000 and above cataracts and IOLs)   Dr Wu Sheng-Quan *Xinjiang, PRC*

1997

- **Certificate of Achievement**   Dr Cai Jing Hong *Xiamen, PRC*
  (1,000 and above cataracts and IOLs)   Dr Wang Hong Gang *Xiamen, PRC*

- **Certificate of Achievement**   Dr Tang Shu Jing *Xiamen, PRC*
  (6,000 anaesthetic procedure for cataract / IOL surgeries)

1999

- **Distinguished Achievement Award** *(5,000 and above cataracts and IOLs)*
  - 10,000   Prof Hong Rong Zhao *Xiamen, PRC*
  - 5,000   Dr Sun Hui-Min *Tianjin, PRC*
  - 5,000   Dr Zhang Hong *Tianjin, PRC*
  - 5,000   Dr Ji Jian *Tianjin PRC*
  - 5,000   Dr Li Xue-Xi *Fujian, PRC*

- **Certificate of Achievement**
  - 3,000   Dr Tang Xin *Tianjin, PRC*
  - 3,000   Dr Xu Yan-Shan *Tianjin, PRC*
  - 2,000   Dr Zhao Shao-Zhen *Tianjin, PRC*
  - 2,000   Dr Wang Zhong-Yi *Liao Ning Province, PRC*
  - 2,000   Dr Zhang Ming-zhi *Xiamen, PRC*
  - 2,000   Dr Wu Guo-Ji *Xiamen, PRC*
  - 1,000   Dr Yang Pei Fei *Fujian, PRC*
  - 1,000   Dr Wu Hu Ping *Xiamen, PRC*

Chapter 12

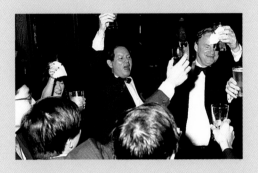

Epilogue

"Towards a glorious future for ophthalmology."

Chapter 12

Epilogue:
The Glorious Future of
Ophthalmology

The 21st century may see the revival of the glorious years of ophthal-mology, when the citizens of the world will enjoy the wonders of modern eye-care.

The 21st century heralds exciting global developments. Frank and open exchange must be fostered between world organisations and leaders in ophthalmology. It is only when we approach these challenges with an open mind that the citizens of the world can enjoy the wonders of modern eye-care.

It is clear that cataract, glaucoma and diabetic retinopathy will be the major causes of blindness. The treatment of such conditions requires the expertise of competent, ethical and committed eye surgeons. Their active role in global blindness-prevention programmes is crucial.

We must turn to Professor Yuan Jia-Qin as a role model in ophthal-mology. The spectacular success of the Tianjin Centre, despite 10 years of difficulties and problems, deserves special mention. Professor Yuan's leadership role in coordinating the centre's programmes, with the help

Towards Glorious Years for Medicine in the 21st Century

The 21st century will usher in the age of "people power". All around the world, including developing countries like Indonesia and the Philippines, citizens are clamouring for their rights. Patients are no exception. They too are demanding the best and the most affordable medical services. Will governments and doctors be able to meet their demands?

"When a nation prospers and begins to embrace the joy of life, it would be unwise to think its citizens would not demand the wonders of modern medicine. There must, of course, be cost restraint, but this is different from simply lowering costs at the risk of lowering quality."

Despite the problems doctors are facing — patients' rising expectations; the proliferation of costly, high technology; escalating health care costs — and which they will continue to face, I am confident that the glorious years of the medical profession will be revived.

The glorious years in the 1950s and 1960s were the most productive and scintillating period for medical science. This was the era of spectacular scientific advances: the discovery of penicillin was swiftly followed by streptomycin for tuberculosis. Preventive measures against polio came next, and were soon out-shone by organ transplantation of the eyes, kidneys, liver and heart.

These advances and more generated waves of public enthusiasm: doctors worldwide were apotheosized to demigod status, parents urged their children to pursue medicine and mothers hoped that their daughters would marry doctors. For the medical profession, this was truly its "Golden Age".

Yet the reputation of doctors has lately seen an insidious decline. More sophisticated patients' expectations, escalating health costs, exorbitant high technology and the dramatic rise in iatrogenic diseases — diseases which developed as a result of treatment - especially the horrors of thalidomide, have cast doubts on scientific progress at a time when human rights — including patients' rights — are gaining prominence.

Medical reforms, especially in the management of patients' desires and expectations, must be effected before medical practitioners can regain the trust and respect of the public. To strengthen the doctor-patient relationship, doctors should be transparent whilst respecting their patients' confidentiality. Ensuring transparency in medical practice would entail surgical outcome evaluation. The outcome should be made available for independent evaluation. This is a clear way of establishing trust between patients and surgeons. The question is: how can surgical outcome be measured effectively and accurately? Indeed, outcome evaluation will be a major concern of doctors in the 21st century.

Next, there must also be reforms in the doctor-doctor relationship. In 1988, Professor Yeoh Ghim Seng, the late Professor of Surgery at the National University of Singapore, expressed deep concern over the self-interest and fear of competition amongst doctors. He also singled out the envy of doctors — the envy of their colleagues who have done well or have excelled in their fields - for criticism. For the medical profession to shine forth in the 21st century, such egotistic individualism should be eradicated and replaced by recognition and praise for professional excellence.

I appeal to the leaders of governments and all doctors to introduce medical reforms, insist on outcome evaluation, control increasing costs, recognise and pursue excellence. Let us, in the 21st century, embrace the wonders of modern medicine and with it, spread the joy of life and happiness to everyone, everywhere. ✢

Adapted from Editorial, Asia-Pacific Journal of Ophthalmology, Vol. 11 No. 4, 1999

of distinguished individuals from different countries, establishes her firmly as the ophthalmic surgeon of the 20th century. If, in the 21st century, the world can nurture leaders like Professor Yuan, then our mission of sight and vision for the world in the year 2020 can be achieved.

For eye surgeons who have not worked in the rural areas of developing nations where the neglected blind are burdened with poverty, ignorance and misery, and where facilities are primitive, they need to sit back and re-examine the principles that have elevated the medical profession to one of honour and high esteem.

Every eye surgeon needs to reflect, "What have I done with my life — have I used my skills to help restore vision to the millions blinded from cataract? Have I used my talents to help the millions afflicted with other vision-threatening eye diseases?"

Eye surgeons of the world, a grave responsibility has been thrust on you. The need for quality eye-care and the battle against mass blindness calls for your valuable professional skills — the citizens of the world depend on you to provide them with their precious vision. You are the beacons of the 21st century. ✳

Appendices

Appendix A

*Supporters and Volunteers from the
World Eye Surgeons Society
(WORLDEYES)*

Afghanistan KAMAL Ziaullah **Algeria** ZEHANI Lamine, **Argentina** SCATTINI Fernando Jorge, EDUARDO Albesi, DOARTERO Carlos M, MALBRAN Enrique S., SARAVIA Mario J, URRETS-ZAVALIA A, CANCERES Gerardo, GUERRERO Josa, **Australia** BILLSON Frank A, COSTER Douglas, TAYLOR Hugh R, CONSTABLE Ian, TAMBLYN D M, LIVINGSTONE-MOLLER Elizabeth, BOOTH Frances, LAM, GODFREY K, COWLE Joffre B, SULLIVAN Lawrence, GRAHAM Peter, SPRING Thomas, GILLIES W E, MULLINS Michael, COOPER Peter, BANASIAK Therese, CAINS Stephen, NICOLL Alan, HERRING Mathew, Frank MARTIN **Austria** EVA Reich phil. Margarete, NEPP Johannes, GABOR Rado, WALTER Richard, RICHARD Waltersdorfer, WIDDER Wolfgang, MÜLLER Elisabeth, MENAPACE Rupert Bahrain, **Bahrain** GHOSH Tarak, **Bangladesh** HUSAIN Rabiul, RAHMAN A. H. Syedur, KHAN Afzal, HUQ Faziul, SHAHID Hassan, RAHMAN Mahbubar, ISLAM Maksudul, KUTUBI Osman Shaheed, AFTAB-VZ-ZAMAN Q M, HYDER Rashid, PINTU Saifuddin Ahmmed, AHMED Sharfuddin, ISLAM Shariful, KHALED Zafar, ISLAM Mahbubul, Matin M A, TARIQ Saifuddin Mohammed, MULLICK Md. Shamsul Hoque, AHMED Shamsuddin, KABIR Md. Humayun **Barbados** KAZI Mohammed A, **Belgium** DEMAN Christian, VAN OYE Rafael, LEYS Anita, VAN LAETHEM Jean, WIJAYA Jusuf, MESTDAGH Christa, ROMMEL Joseph, **Belarus** BIRICH Tamara, IMSHENETSKAYA Tatyana, SAVICH Andrei **Brazil** LIMA Jorge Eldo Silva, DE MENDONCA Benicio Dini, FRANCKOWIAK Stephen Quiroz, ZINSLY Bolivar, SCHEUERMANIN Humberio, MAY Luiz Alberto, TOZATTI Marra SV, JOSE Newton Kara, AVLER Paulo Edvardo, NEVE'S Renato, MARCIA Tartarella, VAN BAAK Alfred, DINIZ Alcides, VIEIRA C, POROIRA Gilborpo L, OLIVALVES Edilberto, **Brunei Darussalam** JOSHI Nayan, **Bulgaria** GOUGHTCHKOVA, KOEV Krassimir, VASSILEVA Petja, CHRISTOVA Rouska, ATANASOVA Blaga Chilova, KOEVA Silvia, MICHEVA Aneta, NAKOWA Anastasia, KOEV Krassimir, LOLOVA Rossitza, ATANASSOV Marin, PETKOVA Natalia, MADJAROVA Ludmila, APOSTOLOV Valentin, **Canada** STEIN Harold, TENCATE Adraian G, TOWNSEND Anthony L, Athanasius RO, ABDEEN Az, PIROUZKAR Behrouz, LEWIS David, ROOTMAN David, LEE Dickson, JOHNSON Ernest A, BEIKO G H H, SAPP G, TAYLOR Garth A, FITTERMAN HN, GOEL Jai NI, MILLER James, SHIN John, KOZ Katherine Deanna, BRIERLEY Lawrence, PIERRE M F Jean, MURPHY Madeleine Hay, ZAHARIA Marian A, KIRKER Merv, HUSSEIN Naushad, COURTRIGHT Paul, MORGAN Rod A, THOMAS Roger, JANS Ronald G, DE SOUZA S, WEINSTOCK S Joseph, RABINOVITCH T, HUNTER W S, MACRAE William G, HALEY Gladys, FARRELL Margaret, CHAM Chuan, SLYVIE Quellet, BRAGA-MELE R, STEVENSON Robert, STEVENSON Heddys, DUBORD Paul, DEMERS Jean Paul, **Columbia** RESHEF Daniel S, **Croatia** FETT Mijo, GRGIC Roza, ROBERT S, VOJNIKOVIC Bozo, SLEZAK Zlatko, **Cuba** AGVIAR Lazgro Perez, TORRES Marcelino Rio, FERRER Olivia Montesino, OBEL GARCIA BAEZ Rodobaldo, CASTRO MESTRE Angel, **Cyprus** ELIA Elias, **Czech Republic** PASTA Jiri, VLADINIR Beran, BAARTOS Dusan, CHOLEVA Martin, SARKA Pitrova, PAVEL Rozsival, PITROVA Sarka, RUZIKOVA Eva, NOVAKOVA Daniela, SURCEK Peter, **Egypt** ALI Ahmed Tawfik, SEWELAM Ashnaf, GALEN Hesham, HUSSEIN Hussein Ali, HANNA Lucy Sharfik, ZAHRA Wadid, EL-LAKKANY Rasheed, EL-MASSRY Ahmed, GOMAA Anhar, HUSSEIN Faten, OSMAN Ahmed, GOMAA Said, SABRY Nabeel, ELSAHN M, EL ZAWAWI Alaa, EL HABROUK Mohamed **Finland** LEIKOLA Johannes, VIHANNINJOKI Kyosil, PAJARI Seppo, PARSSINEU Olavi, BLOMSTER Leif, BLOMSTER Hillevi, DOLGATOVA Ljudmila, JANES Silvi, ZOLOTOROVA Anna, HARTIKAINEN Jouko, Tarkkanen Ahti, Uusitalo Risto J, **France** SARAUX Henry, LOIC-PIERRE Garraud, CLAUDE Benhamou, DENNULI Denis, HOSTYN

Patrick, TRONG Than, CHERON Michel, ISABELLE Meunier, VINCENT Jean Patrick, CHAINE Gilles, SOURDILLE Philippe, WEISER Marc **Georgia** BERADZE Iva, GOLOVACHEV Oleg, OMIADZE Michael, **Germany** PAUST Karsten, KUS M, KNORZ Michael, NEUHANN Thomas F., MORCHER K, **Ghana** NTIM-AMPONSAH CT **Greece** PAPADIMITRIOW Spvros, JOHN Katsimpris, GIAMOURI Maria, INTZES Charalambos, GIANNOULADIS Stilianos, GIANNIKAKIS, PAPAEFTHYMIOU, KATSIMPRIS John, TSOPELAS N., **Hong Kong** HO Patrick, LEUNG Kin Ying, William, WOO Chai Fong, TIAH Toh Ming, LAM Dennis S C, GOLDSCHMIDT Ernest, CHENG George P M, HUI Siu Ping, LIU King Yu, CHOR Michael Fatt Tse, CHAN Pauline Po Chun, KWOK Raymond Kay Tse, TONG Patrick Pak Chuen, **Hungary** FUTO Gabor, NEMETH Janos, LAJES Kolozsvari, DEGI Rosa, PELLE Susanne, A'GNES Szabo, GYETVAI Tama's, HIDASI Vanda, GROSZ Andor, PAPP Andrea, PAMER, Zsuzsanna, PAPP Andras, VASS Peter, SZABO Agnes, DURUCZ Judith, SZIJARTO Zsuzsanna, SALLAI Agnes, CSEKE Istvan, BIRO Zsolt, PELLE Susanna, GYORFFY Istvan, GALLI Lorant, **India** GARG Dinesh, REDDY K Madhukar, VERMA Kishan Baboo, REDDY P Siva, CHANDRA D B, GILL Avtar Singh, WIVEDI Prem Chandra, PRASAD Shyam Sunder, BANSAL Aashish K, AMITAVA Abadan Kman, AGARWAL Agar, RAJENDRA Agarloal, UBOWEJA Anil Kumar, CHATTERJEE Arin, SETHI Arun, AGARWAL Athiya, DUBEY Awadh, BHUSHAN Bharat, SHUKLA Bhushan, MADHIVANAN Chalini, NATH Dharmendra, JILANI F A, NATCHIAR G, VENKATASWAMY G, YADAV H N, DUBAY Harsh, SAINI, J S, THOMAS Jayan, KUMAR K Ratan, MALIK K P S, DUGGAL Kiran, KOTHARI Kulin J, DANDONA Lalit, KHARE M K, SOHANRAJ M, NATARAJAN Madhivanan, CHANDRA Mamesh, SAXENA Manoj, NANDY Manolisa, DESAI N C, AGARWAL N K, AGARWALA Nisheeta, MITTAL Om Parkash, NAMPERUMALSAMY P, SOMDHI Pankat, NARENDRA Patel, THOMAS Philip A, TEJASWI Poorna Chandra, HARDIA Pratap Singh, AKHAORY R K, SRINIVASAN R, MISHRA Rajib Charan, AZAD Rajvardhan, BHARTI S, NATARAJAN S, FERNANDEZ S Tony, THOMAS Saju, NAKHATE Sandeep V, SEN Sanjay, NETHRALAYA Sankara, MULIK Shivaraj, CHAKRAVARTY Somnath, AGARWAL Sunita, TREHAN Vijay Partap, JAGADISH Y S, DESAI Girish, BASU Jyotirmoy, PARANJPE Vijaya, PILLAI K G, JOSHI Shrikant, LION Frans, SHARMA Rajiv, PUNJABI Mahesh, PURI Ashok, JHAMWAR Madusvdan, PATEL Rupande, AGARWAL Anditya, VYAS Prateep, SAMANTA Swapan, CHAUDHRY R M, PASRICHA J K **Indonesia** PT ROHTO LABORATORIES IND, MARSETIO Mardiono, SOEDIRO Hari S., BUDHIASTRA Putu, GHOZI Achmad, SUPARTOTO Agus, SUTRISNO Bamby, BUDIHARDJO, SALAMUN D S M, MAHDI Hariyah M, SIMARMATA M, SUSILA N K Niti, HOETARJO Nannerl, SJAMSOE Soedarman, SUHARDJO, SUPARMAN, GUNAWAN Wasisdi, WIDAGDI S, SOEWONO Wisnujono, SIRLAN Farida, ISKANDAR Abizar, WIDAGDE, TENG K.H, **Iran** MANSOURIFAR Fatemeh, SHAMS Mehdi, AMINOLAH Nikeghbali, MOHEB Davood, SAMIEE Hossein, SALOOR Hossgin, MOHAMMADZADEH G H, ZARRINBAKHSH P, ABOUSAIDE G R, FARAHVASH M S, HASHEMI Hassan, EATESAMI Hassan, LASHRY, CHAMS Hormoz, YAZDANI Ahmad, NILIAHMADABADI, NIKEGHBALI A **Israel** SPIERER Abraham, IRAEL Leshem, BLUMENTHAL M, ZALTZ Mario, BOOCK Marion **Italy** JINGOL Enzo M, CARLEVALE Carlo, MASSIHO Filippello, RENATO Forte, SCUDERI Gianluca, TIBALDI Lorenzo, ACFRES Reibaldi, MARCELLO Santocono, TOGNON Sofia, BARBARA Turrini, MAURIZIO G Uva, PICARDO Vittorio, ANTONIO Lepri, SARNICOLA Vincenzo, DE IORIO Valerio, BACCARA, GALLENGA, BELLO Carlo, PAGANONI Camilllo, GALLENGA Pier E, DOSSI Fabio F **Japan** MATSUI Mizuo, MISHIMA Saiichi, MASUDA Kanjiro, YAMAMOTO Satoru, HOSHIDE Mika, SHIWA Toshihiko, KONNO Yasuhiro, SUZUKI Koji, NAKAJIMA Akira, SATO Tsuyoshi, NAGATA Makoto **Jordan** SIRHAN Nafiz I, YAHYA D Othman A ADAS Fathi A, AYESH Ibrahim, MADANAT Ayman **Kazakhstan** MAMBETOV Ekpin **Kenya** MATHENGE Wanjiku, **Korea** KIM Jae Ho, SANG Wook-Rhee, KIM Wan-Soo, RHEE Sang Wook, **Kuwait** GOSWAMY Subhash **Kyrgyzstan** AKAEVA Mairam D, IMANBACVA Saltanat **Latvia** OIBEDE Mairo, JGOR Solonivatim, VALKOVA Irene, **Lebanon** CHIKHANI Walid, **Libya** HAMUDA Abdulmuhaimen **Lithuania** BAGDONIENE Rasa, BANIULIENE Danguole, SIRAUTIENE Rasa, ULICKIENE Ruta **Malawi** CHIPAMBO M C, CHIRAMBO Moses, **Malaysia** SELVARAJAH S, RAVINDRAN Vijayalekshmy, CHAN Cordelia, CHING Wing Seng, RAMANI Veera, SAAD Ahmad Mt, MAJUMDER Ajit, DAHALAN Alias, TAN Andrew Khian Khoon, AU Mun Kit, PILLAI Balaravi, CHIN Pik Kee, CHOO May May, CHOONG Yean Yaw, KRISHNAN Hari, KIEW Chit Choa, SIDHU Manjit S, MUSADIQ Mohammed, MAJID Mohd Wadzik, MUTHUSAMY P, SINGH Pall, RAMASAMY Rajagordl s/o, SIVARAJ Rajamalika, YEO K C Robert, REDDY S C, SELVI, REDDY T.N. Krishna, Tan Niap Ming, SUBRAYAN Visvaraja, LEE Y C, GHANI Zulkifli Abdul, LEE Seow Yeang, BROHIER William G, THANGASAMY Vasantha Kumar, KONG Dennis, SINGH Sarbjit, TAN Niap Ming, **Malta** JANULA Jan, **Maritius** BAHEMIA A M, **Mexico** ALMADA Julio Martinez, GREENE Irene Olhovich, MEDINA Hector, GOMEZ Jose Antonio Garcia, VALLEJO Miguel Alvaarezy, **Moldava** NOVAC Valeri, GRIBONOSOV Serghey, **Morocco** ABDELOVAHED Ahraovi, **Myanmar** NYUNT Kan, AUNG Mya, AUNG Than, **Nepal** UPADHYAY Madan P, SHRESTHA Jeevan K, SHARMA Anil Kumar, BADHU Badri Prasad, SHARMA Basant Raj, DAHAL Chhabi Raman, POKHREL Ram Prasad, KHADKA Basanta, **New Zealand**

SABISTON David, **Nigeria** OWIE Joe, **Norway** RIISO Dag, GARBORG Herdis, **Oman** ZUTSHI Rajiv, **Pakistan** BAIG Amin Ullah, QAZI Muhammad Azhar, MOHAMMAD Zia, MUMTAZ Raja, KHAN Mohammad Daud, ANKLESARIA H S, AZHAR Jacob Salim, KHAN M Aman, KHAN M Zahoor I, YAQIN Mohammad, SAEED Muhammad, FAROOQ Muhammad Umar, AHMAD Rashid, RAHMAN S Saif-ur, IQBAL Zafar, SHAIKH Ziauddin A, SIDDIQUI G R, ISLAM Ziaul, REHMAN Najeeb-ur, BODLA M Afzal, AHMED Raheed, QURESHI, BUTT Nadeem H, MUKHTAR-AHMED Muhammad, **Papua New Guinea** VERMA Nitin, **Paraguay** QUINTANA Luz Marina, GARCETE Olga **Peru** CONTRERAS Francisco, FRANCKOWIAK Annette Quiroz, **Philippines** LIM Matabai A, GESTUVO Rolando G, FERNANDEZ-SUNTAY Jackie, TAN Roberto C, MARTINEZ Alfredo B, VALDEZ Alma Malabag, DE LEON Anceles, ROMERO B D, MENDOLA Barbara Ann D, RADUL Henson, ARRIBAS Irwin C, BALDERAS Joanne J, GAHOL Luisito, AGULTO Manuel, QUESING Manuel, SANTOG Marcelo F, DOMINGO Marilyn I, RIVERA Mary Katherine, NGM Michael S, SISON Michael, FAJARDO Moises Romeo G, CRUZ Paul D, DOMINGO Perfecto S, YANG Richard S, LEE Rolando B, MILANTE Rollo, SINGSON Roseny Mae C, HENSON Ruben, LIM Ruben Bon Siong, ANG Sammy L, TAN Timothy, C RONGUILLO Yasmymo, BANGERT Kurt, ALIVIA Josephine R, KING Jacqueline H, GALERA Florida S, SANTOS MA Cristina M, VALDEZ MA Victoria, TE-MILANA Kim, REGALA Renato M, ALFONSO Mario Andrew A, RODRIGUEZ Rafael E, LIM Maria Elaine, VERCELES Maria Christina, TIRONA Lorelie B, ACOB Loida, SUGALA Nilo, NAVAL Cosme, ALBORNOZ Rodolfo M, PALANCA-CAPISTRANO Angelita M, HENRY Elnora J, URGEL Joselito D C, LIBRE JR Maximino S, TALEON Rose Janet T, ZERNUDO Zeny Rose B, CASTILLO Irene S, CATACUTAN Amador R, PINEDA Grego K, SAMSON Victorino C, REGALADO Rolando E, GENUINO Estrellita S, ELEVADO Malyn C, TOLENTINO Edwin C, SAY Antonio, MANACO JR Francisco B, SINOLINDING JR Kadil, TORNO Ricardo B, CAPUCHINO-VILLALVA Corazon, PALANOA Lumen R, PEROS-GALAM Remelyn, CORONICA Rolly R, COLL Josephine V MA, URMAZA Santiago G, NANAGAS Juan R, CUSTODIO Joseph T, JORDAN Florencita N, PARAAN Ronaldo A, MANALO JR Francisco B, PRINCIPE Roy Teodoro B, URGEL Mary Joan T, ROASA Ruperto V, **Poland** MOHAMED El Hussein I, STANISLAWA Gierek-Kazicka, EWA Mrvkwa, DOROTA Wygledowska, MOHAMED El-Hussein Mnisy, LAZARCZYK Alina, BERDNARCZYK-MELLER Jadwiga, JUROWSKI Piotr, MUZYKA Maria, ZAJAC-PYTRUS Hanna, SZYMANSKI Andrzej, DE LAVAL Wtodzimierz, BVDZYNSKA-SILDATKE Anna, UJAZDOWSKA Anna, GINTER Matgorzata, HABELA Marek, TURNO-KRECICKA Anna, GIEREK-LAPINSKA Ariadna, **Portugal** LUIS Perira, GAMA Rita, LEONG Chan, ROCHA SOUSA Amandio, VELUDO Maria Joao, MACEDO DOS SANTOS Joao Paulo, CUHNA-VAZ Jose, LEITE Eugenio O, **PR China** HONG Rong Zhao, WU Hu Ping, WU Guo Ji, ZHANG Ming Zhi, HUANG Jia Huang, WANG Qing Ying, LU Jian Hua, ZHU Gang, ZHAO Shao-Zhen, CHEN Wei, YUAN Jia Qin, ZHANG Shu, WANG, P. Tarrno, CHAN Xiang-Hai, CHENG Shi Ming, DING Ke Xi, GU Xun Qing, GUO Hai Ke, HAO Yansheng, HUANG Pei Gang, JI Jian, JIANG You Qin, LAI Zong Bai, LEE Xiao Rong, LI Shaozhen, LI Xue-Xi, LIU Fang Yi, LIU Ya Dong, SHENG Lian Zhu, WANG Qin Mei, XIN Tang, YANG Chun Yan, XU Yan-Shan, ZHANG Hong, ZHANG Lin, ZHANG Zheng Guo, ZHAO Kanxing, ZHOU Yuan Qing, TANG Shu Chen, SUN Hui Min, SHI Wenyong, **Republic of Panama** BOYD Benjamin F, BARRAZA Andres Caballero, **Romania** JURJA Sanda, KIRSTIUK Cristina, PASCARIU Francisca, FLORIAN Dan, PREDOIU Daniela, **Russia** KHVEDELIANI David J, UZUNYAN Julietta G, **Russian Fed** PERSHIN Kirill, MAITCHOUK Iouri, CHLIAPOUJNIKOVA Alina, PASHINOVA Nadezda, TMOYANOVSKY Roman, BRZHESKY Vladimir, DISKALENKO Oleg, AVDEEV Peter Alexejevich, BESSMEZTAY Alexander, SEON-MARTIAL Lynette **Saudi Arabia** SHAMS Abdul Moiz, BADEEB Osama, MCKINNEY J Kevin, AMIN Hosam, ISLAM Sara **Singapore** Singapore Eye Foundation, KOH Adrian, ANG Beng Chong, ANG Chong Lye, LIM Kuang Hui, LOW Cze Hong, TAN Donald, WONG Doric, KHOO Chong Yew, CHEW Paul, YONG Victor, WAI Charity, LIM Arthur S M, TSENG Peter, YEOH Ronald, YEO Kim Teck, AU EONG Kah Guan, AUNG Tin, CHEE Caroline, CHAN Tat Keong, CHAN Wing Kwong, CHUA Ee Chek, CHIANG Currie, SIM Daniel Han Jen, OEN Francis, GOH Swee Heng, HENG Lee Kwang, GOH Jon, KOH Lian Buck, LEE Hung Ming, LIM Li, LIM Tock Han, LOW Siew Ngim, YEO Lynn, PHUA Raymond, TANEJA Sangeeta, HO Tony Kee Wai, YAP Eng Yiat, YAP Soo Keong, LING Yvonne, JAP Aliza Hee Eng, WANG Lee Yuen, SIOW Ka Lin, YEO Liew Soo, WONG Jun Shyan, HO Kok Tong, AMRITH Shantha, TAN Geok Tian, BALAKRISHNAN V, TAN Swan Jeng, LEONG Dominic **Slovac Republic** DOMINOVA Tatiana, KUDLOVA Ludmila, SPIRKOVA Jana, STUBNA Michal, SUCH Marian, VISNANSKY, THOMAS Khia's, PETER Strmer, **Slovenia** PUSNIK Dusan, PRIMOZ Logar, VESELY Trantisew, JURINEC-VAJDA Sonja, RUBIN Ivan, MLINAR Peter, STABUC-SILIH Mirna **South Africa**, GRAEMIGER Roman, LETLAPE Kgost, SEBBI Esmael, MEYER D, EPSTEIN Edward, **Spain** LOPEZ-RAMOS Pedro, ENRIQUE Aleman, CORIHUELA Carlos, TEMPRANDO Jose, AGUIRRE Justo, PINERO Antonio, PARDO MUNOZ Ascension, MENEZO Luis, **Sri Lanka** MENDIS Upali, SEIMON Reggie, SEIMON C R, PILAPIITYA Kasyapa, **Sudan** SULEIMAN Farouk, **Suriname** HILDEGARD H, **Sweden** JAKOBSSAN Gunner, DHIR Meryl, PHILIPSON Bo T, ZETTERSTROM Charlotta,

Switzerland BIJAN Farpour, FLAMMER Josef, STUCCHI Carlo A, **Syria** HABAL, ANTAKI Samir G, **Taiwan** HUI Chun Tai, LEE Ray Fong, HUANG, **Thailand** TEEKHASAENEE Chaiwai, SETHASUOVAN Chanchai, HIRI-O-TAPPA Juthathip, KHANGRANG Noppadol, ROJANAPONGPUN Prin, YAISAWANG Sudarat **The Netherlands** DEUTMAN August F, SMITH Gerard M, PARLEVLIET Len, DEN BOON Mariius, WORST Jan G F, VAN RIJ G, VAN DER POL Bert A E, AALDER-DEENSTRA Victoriene, BUISMAN Nico, BLANKSMA, DRAGT Henk, HENDRATA Khoen, KLEIN POELHUIS Wim, KOESMAN Laura, KOOLE Frank, POL Van Der, LEFEBER Anthony, STILMA Jan, ZAAL Michael, CARENINI Lucia, WINDT C Van Der, KORVER Cornelius, JUNGE J **Trinidad & Tobago** HOSEIN Robin **Turkey** KAYNAK Suleyman, ERGIM Ayfer, GERGI Dilek, TURACLI Erol, TALU Haluk, ELTUTAR Kadir, KEVSER M H, KASKALOGLU Mahmut, PAPILLA MEDICAL LTD, KARADEDE D Sezin, COSAR C Banu, OZEN Yuksel, ALACALI Nilay, BIRINCI Hakki, ARITURK Nursen, GUL KOCAK ALTINTAS Ayse, KOCAK Inci, GUVEN Dilek, OKKA Mehmet, YALAZ Muslim, OZTURK Faruk, YAZAR Zeliha, KURT Emin, KARADENIZ, GENC Selim **UK** RICE Noel S, WATSON Peter G, FOULDS Wallace S, KLEANTHOUS Luke, ROSEN Paul H, PRASAD Somdutt, CHANDRA Girish, HAROON M Am, MOSS David, WHILE A, RAHMAN Abdur, DAMATO Bertil, IMAFIDON Chris, FIBERESIMA D Denni, INFELD David A, GORDON N Dutton, MACKINTOSH Graeme, KWAKH Jeffery, THOMSITT John, WU John, KYLE Peter Mcleod, PERCIVEL Piers, MURRAY Stephen, PITTS John, ROSEN Emanuel S, STEVENS Susan M, RICH Walter, AL-IBRAHIM Jalil, AL-KHAIER Ayman, KHAN Khalid, MATHEN George, NYLANDER Arthur, BLACK Peter, AJEWOLE Olutunde, NYLANDER A G E, MAKAR I H, SANDRAMOULI S, TAYLOR Bob, **Ukraine** BOITCHUK Irina M, LOGAY Ivan M, WU Li Jing, BOBROVA Nadejda F, IVANOVA Nana, PETRUNYA Andrey, POLOUNINE Guennadi, LIJUIP W, KOGAN B, **USA** SOMMER Alfred, SHAH Harshad G, HOLZINGER Karl A, SHOFNER Stewart, BROWN Harry S, USSA Fernando, CATE Adrian G Ten, AHMAD Afzal, SIMJEE Aisha, JONES Alan C, FISHERMAN B, LINDER Barry J, KWAN Benjamin, SMITH Bruce, KOLLARITS Carol R, BURNS Charlotte A, GIRKIN Chris, SLADE Clifton, DAVIS Dale, KROWTZ Dan, COOK David W, WILSON Doug R, SHORE Doug, COT LIER Edward, KIM Edward W, PAYDAR Frashid, NEWMAN Frederic, CHIN George N, METZ Gerald A, PREECS Gordon R, ARANGO Gustauo, WANG H S, NEALIS Henry J, MAISEI James M, FREEMAN Jerre Minor, JERNIGAN Jerry M, BELADO John, FLAXEL John, WRIGHT John, BUKA Jonathan, KHORRAM K David, COHEN Kenneth L, KHAN Khalid Latif, PAH Lawrence, ORTICIO R N Lily P, FELDGOISE Louis T, SANTANGOLD Maura, LUNTZ Maurice H, HENRY Max A, ROSE Michael R, KINI Mohandas, LONGDUN Nathan, LEWIS Norman, CHRISTY Norval E, CAVLSON Paul, BRAZIS Peter, GONZALEZ-SIRIT Rafael, GOULSTON Ralph N, ROSENQUIST Robert C, JONES Robert, TREFT Robert, DEWIN Sanjeen, SIBAYAN Santiago Antonio B, SHERIDAN Selma J, RABIN Sheldon, BERNIE Stephan, THOMS Susan, DICKINSON Thomas J, STILES William, KEATES Edwin U, FIDUCCIA Frank S, NARPER John Y, ALLARAKHIA Liaquat, PIECUCH Brian, GOINS Gary D, BAKOS Jim, ALEPPO Joseph A, AYLOO Kausalya, BERGEY Ray M, BROWN Ballie R, SHAN Gao, SIEPSER Steven B, HARLEY II William W, FARCI Fernando, SCHULTZ Gerald, TABA Katia, WARREN Keith, HIRSCHMAN Henry, RICH Alan M, KHORRAM K David, FRYCZKOWSKI Andy, BURNSTEIN Alan, KHAN Hamza N, NATHAN Francis, O'DAY David G, QIUSHI Ren, SAWYER Ralph A, BROWN David, HIRSCHMAN Henry, MICHELIS Mary Kay, **Venezuela** RIVAS Armando, BERMUZEL Ahaya, MILGROM B, ALEXIDZE Alexander, **Vietnam** VU Tue Khanh, LAN Le Ngoc, CUNG Le Xuan, HOANG Thi Minh Chau, VAN Pham My Khanh **Yugoslavia Rep** MARJANOVIC Sima, KONTIC Djordje, ALEKSIC Petar, **Zambia** SHARMA M K **Zimbabwe** D'SOUZA Roy Agnel, GURAMATUNHU Solomon ✳

Appendix B

The Challenge of Glaucoma

Arthur S M Lim, Singapore

A bewildering array of medical technology and scientific advances awaits us in the 21st century. Although we have made significant inroads into cataract and diabetic retinopathy, glaucoma remains an enigma.

Of these major blinding conditions, especially in developing countries, cataract blindness will be resolved in 20 years. Implant surgery restores normal vision to the patient while the problem remains that of organisation. For a model, we should refer to the International Intraocular Implant Training Centre in Tianjin, China, where 2,250 eye surgeons have been trained and normal vision has been restored to 120,000 blind cataract patients with low-cost extracapsular cataract extraction and lens implantation.[1] This centre has paved the way for the establishment of similar centres around the developing world.

As far as diabetic retinopathy is concerned, ophthalmologists have the grave responsibility of making sure that blindness is controlled in the early stages with screening, especially since early treatment with laser photocoagulation is known to prevent blindness in 90% of carefully treated patients.[2] With effective organisation, most patients with diabetic retinopathy will not suffer severe visual loss or blindness.

Editorial, Joint Millennium Issue of the Asian Journal of Ophthalmology and the Asia-Pacific Journal of Ophthalmology, January 2000

In contrast, despite decades of research and debate, most problems associated with open angle glaucoma require further clarification. We do not fully understand the condition; the epidemiology is confusing. Even its definition eludes us. For these reasons, glaucoma will emerge as the most challenging discipline of the 21st century.

We are fortunately more knowledgeable about angle closure glaucoma. The condition is mechanical and is based on the anatomical occlusion of a normal but narrow filtrating angle by the iris and, depending on the extent and rapidity of the occlusion, it can present clinically as acute, sub-acute, or chronic angle closure glaucoma.

It has been known for many years that angle closure glaucoma is more common in Asians, whereas amongst Caucasians, open angle glaucoma is more common. More specifically, this epidemiological pattern is found mainly in Chinese populations, but not in other Asians.

Why is angle closure glaucoma more common among Chinese people? Does it result from intrinsic differences between Chinese and Caucasians? What is the impact of these differences on clinical practice?

No one is certain why angle closure glaucoma is more common in Chinese people, but evidence suggests that it is due to the anatomical structure of the eye; a smaller eye with a shallow anterior chamber and a narrow filtrating angle. Dim lighting or reading will dilate the pupil and increase the pupillary block and iris bombe, causing closure of the narrow filtrating angle, which can trigger off acute angle closure glaucoma. In addition, acute glaucoma is more severe in Chinese populations and frequently requires trabeculectomy to control the increased pressure.[3,4]

The effectiveness of laser in angle closure glaucoma is different for Caucasians and Chinese. It has been known for some time that YAG laser is effective for the thin blue iris of Caucasians, but is far less effective in the thick brown iris of Chinese eyes, for whom a combination of Argon laser with the YAG appears to be the most effective approach.

An important use of laser is to apply contraction laser burns at the iris periphery, a procedure known as iridoplasty. The brown iris can be made to contract by use of Argon laser with power of approximately 500 mW, diameter of 250 micron and time of 0.50 seconds. These contractions of the iris are of particular value in acute angle closure glaucoma — the iris is pulled away from the angle which opens up the angle, and the high intraocular pressure from acute glaucoma can be rapidly and effectively lowered. Laser is especially valuable in situations where medication has failed to reduce the pressure; for example, in acute glaucoma. Iridoplasty, unfortunately, is not without complications. In addition, its effectiveness is usually temporary and many eyes will still require a peripheral iridotomy, trabeculectomy, or cataract surgery. In spite of the complications, iridoplasty will be more commonly used worldwide as it is an effective procedure in the treatment of angle closure glaucoma.[5]

The racial difference makes it likely that screening of elderly Chinese women for angle closure glaucoma will become important as it is cost-effective to screen this select group.[6]

When progression of angle closure glaucoma is slow and the raised pressure insidious, chronic angle closure glaucoma presents as open angle glaucoma, and clinically, they are indistinguishable except with gonioscopy. It is therefore essential to remember, especially for Chinese patients, that all patients diagnosed with chronic open angle glaucoma should have their angles evaluated.

During the past decades, our knowledge about open angle glaucoma has not significantly advanced. Today, we are not even certain of the desired level of intraocular pressure for glaucoma patients. At one stage, it was 22 mm Hg, although some have argued that each eye with glaucoma has a different desirable pressure, while in some countries, especially Japan, where normal pressure glaucoma is common, there are indications that high pressure is not the only risk factor in glaucoma.

Numerous research papers have been presented on visual field studies using different computer programmes. Disadvantages of these tests are that they are all subjective (dependent on the patient's response), and that a firm decision on the progress of the field defect cannot not be made until tests have been repeated several times.

In addition, there are conflicting views on the observations of the optic disc cup. When is it pathological and how should it be recorded? It is clear that the stereo disc record is important and should be performed for all patients with glaucoma. However, the more expensive, complex laser imaging and similar techniques of recording the optic disc cup are not cost-effective; at the present moment, they are used mainly for research purposes. Yet, because open angle glaucoma will become increasingly important, we can only hope that more effective equipment for a precise measurement of the optic disc cup will become cheaper.

Pathology in open angle glaucoma, the changes in the trabecular meshwork, and the reasons why the optic disc becomes damaged — and whether this is due to a defective vascular supply or some other factors — remain uncertain despite years of molecular biology studies and millions of dollars spent on glaucoma research. More recently, genetics and interference with genes have offered the possibility of more significant advances.

Numerous new eye drops are being introduced every few months; some have become popular partly because they can lower intraocular pressure more effectively and hopefully, prevent blindness. They are marketed by profit-making organisations although this is not unusual in a free market economy where companies aggressively promote their products.

While we appreciate these advances, careful studies should be done on the cost-effectiveness of the eye drops, as well as their real long-term value to patients with glaucoma throughout the world. The prostaglandin latanoprost appears to be more effective in its pressure-lowering effect, although recent studies suggest that medication which protects the optic nerve disc from damage may be the answer for open angle glaucoma.[7]

Trabeculectomy, touted as a great advance, fails because of scarring in many cases. Although 5-fluorouracil and mitomycin-C can delay scarring, their positive effects are counter balanced by possible complications from defective wound healing as well as infection (endophthalmitis can rapidly blind the eye).[7] When is it justified to operate on 1-eyed patients? After all, chronic glaucoma takes years to blind the typical patient, sometimes even beyond his lifespan, whereas it takes only a few days to inflict blindness with surgery. This explains why several eminent international experts in glaucoma have publicly stated that patients can be worse off following surgery.

Indeed, experienced clinicians are important in the management of complex glaucoma and should balance the enthusiasm for short-term procedures and technology with the considerations for long-term management. As Epstein has stated, *"The fields of glaucoma are littered with relics of short-term enthusiasms for certain procedures and techniques."*[8]

Of all the fascinating challenges we will confront in the 21st century, glaucoma promises to be the most intriguing. Young ophthalmologists eager to face the challenges of ophthalmology in the new millennium, will find themselves drawn to the study, management, and surgery of glaucoma. As glaucoma is not only the affliction of individuals, but also a leading cause of world blindness, they will find themselves embarking on an exciting and profitable odyssey of global significance. ✳

References

1. Lim ASM. Eye surgeons – seize the opportunity. Am J Ophthalmol 1996;122:571-573.

2. Blankenship GW. Fifteen-year argon laser and xenon photocoagulation results of Bascom Palmer Eye Institute's patients participating in the diabetic retinopthy study. Ophthalmology 1991;98:125-128.

3. Lowe RF, Lim ASM. Clinical pathology. In Primary Angle Closure Glaucoma. Singapore: PG publishing, 1989;II:20.

4. Lim ASM. Primary angle closure glaucoma in Singapore. Aust J Ophthalmol 1979; 7:23-30.

5. Lim ASM, Tan A, Chew P, et al. Laser iridoplasty in the treatment of severe acute angle closure glaucoma. Int Ophthalmol 1993;17:33-36.

6. Seah S, Foster PJ, Chew PTK, et al. Incidence of acute primary angle-closure glaucoma in Singapore. Arch Ophthalmol 1997;115:1436-1440.

7. Aung T, Wong HT, Chee CY, et al. Comparison of the intraocular pressure-lowering effect of latanoprost and timolol in patients with chronic angle closure glaucoma. A randomised double-masked study. Annual Meeting of the Association for Research in Vision and Ophthalmology (ARVO), May 9-14, 1999, Florida, USA.

8. Epstein DL. Introduction. In Epstein DL, Allingham RR, Schuman JS (eds), Chandler and Grant's Glaucoma. 4th ed. Baltimore: Williams & Wilkins, 1997;I:3.

Appendix C

References

Chapter 2: "I Want to See"

1. Woods AC. The adjustment to aphakia. Am J Ophthalmol. 1952;35:118-22.

2. Sommer A. Obstacles and Opportunities: New Frontiers in Ophthalmology: Proceedings of the XXVIICO, March 1990. New York: Elsevier Science Inc. 1990:18-24.

3. Taylor HR. Public health perspective for cataract surgery. Proceedings of the 2nd International Ophthalmologic Conference, July 1995 Beijing.

4. Lim ASM. Vision for the World. Singapore: World Scientific Publishing Co Ltd.1996: 27-8.

5. Lim ASM. Eye surgeons' essential role in cataract blindness. Proceedings of the 16th Congress of the Asia Pacific Academy of Ophthalmology, March 1997 Kathmandu.

6. Lim ASM. Eye surgeons: Seize the opportunity. Am J Ophthalmol. 1996;122:571-3.

7. Lim ASM. Human Right to Normal Vision. Singapore: World Scientific Publishing Co Ltd. 1997.

Chapter 6: "Eye Surgeons – Seize the Opportunity"

1. Lim ASM. Vision for the world. Singapore: World Scientific Publishing Co. Ltd., 1996:v.

2. Lim ASM. Impact of technology on mass blindness in Asia. Jpn J Ophthalmol 1987; 31:375-83.

3. Kahn H. Towards the next 200 years. New York: Morrow and Co., 1976:1.

4. Lim ASM. Vision for the world. Singapore: World Scientific Publishing Co. Ltd., 1996:35.

5. World Health Organisation. Eleventh Annual Meeting of the WHO Programme Advisory Group on the Prevention of Blindness: New Delhi, India, February 28 to March 3, 1995. Geneva, Switzerland: World Health Organisation, 1995.

Chapter 10: "The Dilemma of Ophthalmic Changes Spreads to Asia"

1. Watts G. Looking to the future. In: Roy Porter, editor. Cambridge illustrated history of medicine. Cambridge: Cambridge University Press, 1998:357.

2. Lim ASM. Vision for the world: a solution to the major world medical problem of mass blindness. Singapore: World Scientific Publishing Co, 1996.

3. Toffler A. The third wave. London: Pan Books, in Association with Collins, 1981.

Appendix D

Acknowledgments

I am particularly indebted to my wife, Mrs Arthur Lim, for her scrupulous editing and for joining me in my vision against cataract blindness.

Dr Ang Beng Chong, my able and dedicated partner and his wife, Dr Su Hong Hai, and the nursing staff led by Sister Peck Chye Fong for supporting my efforts so strongly, at a time when the use of implant was uncertain. The late Mr Chan Seng Poh and his daughter, Ms Chan Poh Choo for their generous donations and Ms Charity Wai for her continued efforts in the communication and administration of the activities.

The coordination and fluency of the text is made possible through the efforts of Ms Julie Goh and Ms Leona Lo.

To Professor Joaquin Barraquer, Spain, I express my gratitude for his permission to reproduce the slides; Professor Yuan Jia-Qin, PRC, and Professor Hong Rong-Zhao, PRC, for their permission to reproduce various pictorials and newspaper articles; the American Journal of Ophthalmology, Hong Kong Journal of Ophthalmology, Asian Journal of Ophthalmology and the Asia-Pacific Journal of Ophthalmology for their permission to reproduce the editorials.

I have Jeffrey Goh from SinKho Advertising and Design to thank for the design and visual layout support.

I would also like to thank Alcon for their generous sponsorship of this book. ✳